Meal Plan on a Budget

A 30-days fantastic cookbook of meal prep for beginners. 100+ recipes for planning your family meals. Save your time and value your money!

Author : **Eric Carrie**

INTRODUCTION

Did you realize that you can cook and heat on one day and make suppers that will sustain your family for a month? This inexorably well-known type of transport line cooking isn't as troublesome as it sounds, and can really be a great deal of fun. You will figure out how to utilize your cooler, broiler, microwave, barbecue, and moderate cooker to cook and store delectable, sound suppers that you can simply haul out and warm for breakfast, lunch, or supper in minutes. Envision having the weight of arranging, shopping, cooking, and serving supper each and every day lifted from your shoulders—it's an unimaginable inclination.

This kind of cooking can be adjusted to any food. Do you adore Mexican nourishment? You can make and stop a base of meat and vegetables that can be utilized for enchiladas, tacos, burritos, taco plate of mixed greens, Mexican pizza, fajitas, and Tex-Mex soups and stews.

Is your family snared on Italian cooking? A base of ground meat can be utilized for spaghetti, cannelloni, manicotti, and lasagna. The varieties are practically perpetual!

There are a couple of approaches to handle making dinners for a month. You can cook triple bunches of your most loved plans and stop them in dinner size compartments; you can cook ten to thirty individual plans and stop them; or you can purchase a huge amount of meats and fixings, cook a major bunch of starter nourishments, and after that make loads of various meals and dishes from the starter clump.

Furthermore, did you realize you can heat and stop breads, treats, bars, cakes, and different pastries?

Putting away these nourishments implies you will consistently be readied when the organization drops in out of the blue, and you will be prepared for any occasion feast or family festivity.

You'll set aside cash since you can purchase what's unique in your grocery store and utilize each piece.

What's more, there's actually no preferable inclination over realizing your cooler is loaded with enough nourishment to sustain your family for a month. Once-a-month cooking is extraordinary compared to other timesavers in the kitchen.

You can likewise be the closest companion and neighbor when you are a fan of once-a-month cooking.

At whatever point life ends up hard for somebody you know, you can offer the most magnificent present: a hot, solid, delectable home-prepared dinner immediately.

Likely the most significant reward of this cooking technique is this: getting ready crisp, delectable dinners for your family encourage them to carry on with a solid way of life. You won't need to arrange takeout nourishments or rely upon costly drive-through eateries with their sodium-stacked, high-fat food sources. Cooking solid nourishments for yourself and your family is an approach to make everybody feel very much bolstered and thought about. So how about we begin on the experience of The Everything® Meals for a Month Cookbook!

Contents

CHAPTER ONE

FROZEN FOOD BASICS

If you are new to once-a-month cooking, the procedure may appear to be overpowering. Simply approach it slowly and carefully. With each progression you complete, your certainty will develop. Before you start, there are a few things you have to think about solidifying nourishment.

All nourishment is comprised of live cells, which are little building squares. These cells contain catalysts, water, protein, and different synthetic concoctions that respond with air and water to steadily cause weakening, known as ruining, as the nourishment ages. At the point when nourishment is solidified, the elements of cells delayed down drastically; this jam the nourishment. Solidifying can't improve the nature of nourishment; it essentially holds it at the quality it was when solidified. Synthetic concoctions in the nourishment will, in any case, be dynamic notwithstanding during the solidified state, despite the fact that this movement is significantly decreased.

There are a few factors in nourishment that influence the solidifying procedure. Here's a short review of these realities so you can benefit from your cooler and this technique for cooking.

Microscopic organisms and Molds

Microscopic organisms and molds are available all over, even on the nourishment we eat. Solidifying stops the development of microscopic organisms and shape on nourishments; be that as it may, when the nourishment is defrosted, these microorganisms will start to develop once more. That is the reason it is so critical to defrost nourishments in the fridge rather than at room temperature. Bacterial action is as yet smothered exposed to the harsh elements demeanor of the refrigerator. Cooking obliterates microbes and molds, so it's essential to appropriately and altogether warm solidified nourishment before eating it.

Freezer Burn

A freezer is a threatening spot. Nourishments that are not appropriately bundled for the freezer will turn into harmed rapidly. Freezer burn is the most well-known issue of the solidifying procedure. It's just the lack of hydration of nourishment. At the point when nourishment is inappropriately wrapped, the dry condition of the freezer draws off dampness as the nourishment solidifies. This harms cells in the nourishment and results in dry, hard fixes that won't return to the hydrated state notwithstanding when defrosted. Nourishment that is influenced by cooler consume isn't perilous to eat, yet it will be extreme and need enhance. If solitary a modest quantity of nourishment is influenced by freezer burn, you can basically remove that region and heat and eat the rest. In the event that there is freezer burn over a huge territory of the nourishment, be that as it may, toss it out; the taste and surface will be undermined.

Stews, soups, and other fluid nourishments that have been influenced by cooler consume might be spared. These normally fluid nourishments can ingest the harm brought about by the lack of hydration when warmed. Add ¼ cup water to the dish when warming, and blend delicately.

To avoid freezer burn, wrap nourishments firmly. Likewise, be certain the provisions you buy to wrap and store your nourishment are explicitly created for the cooler condition.

Enzymes and Oxidation

Enzymes that are normally present in nourishment cause changes in shading, flavor, and surface. Enzymatic procedures don't stop when nourishment is solidified, despite the fact that they do back off. A few nourishments, especially foods grown from the ground, should be whitened or quickly cooked before solidifying to incapacitate these catalysts.

Cells are finished bundles with films that control water and air trade. Whenever cells have been harmed (cut, slashed, or torn) by getting ready or preparing the nourishment, air consolidates with compounds inside the cells. This procedure is called enzymatic oxidation, and it stains nourishment and changes flavors. Fats in meat can end up malodorous. The shade of foods grown from the ground can end up dull and boring. Solidifying limits this procedure, and you can help by expelling however much air as could reasonably be expected from the nourishment when bundling it. Additionally, when you are getting ready natural products for the cooler, cover the cut surfaces with an acidic fluid-like lemon juice or an ascorbic corrosive answer for stoppage the oxidation procedure.

Get the Air Out

Air is the adversary when you're frosty nourishments! Evacuate however much air as could be expected when wrapping.

When you bundle nourishment, push down on the holder to dispose of abundance air. You can utilize a drinking straw to coax let some circulation into before fixing the bundle. Be that as it may, fluid things, for example, soups and stews need a limited quantity of room, called headspace, in the holder to consider extension during solidifying. Leave ½ inch of headspace in these holders so the top doesn't fly off when the nourishment grows as it solidifies.

The Freezer(s)

You might need to put resources into an independent chest cooler on the off chance that you are going to make this sort of cooking some portion of your life. The cooler that is a piece of your fridge can likewise be utilized as long as it isn't overstuffed with nourishment.

When adding new bundles of nourishment to your freezer, attempt to put them in the base of the cooler or against the sides. These are the coldest pieces of the cooler, so the nourishment will solidify all the more rapidly without raising the inward temperature.

Utilize a freezer thermometer to ensure that your cooler is at a temperature of 0°F or lower before you stock it with nourishment. If that conceivable, turn your freezer to–10°F when you include nourishment. At the point when the nourishment is solidified strong, you can turn the temperature back to 0°F.

If you have an additional independent freezer, store it in the storm cellar or the coolest piece of your home.

At that point, if the power goes off, the surrounding air temperature will keep the temperature inside the cooler for a more drawn out timeframe. In the event that the power goes off, keep the cooler shut. You might need to envelop it by covers or towels to help protect it and hold the temperature down. Most independent coolers will remain at 0°F or less for twenty-four to thirty hours without power.

Many independent freezer should be defrosted each six to a year. Adhere to producer's directions for defrosting. While defrosting your freezer, dispose of bundles that are over a year old and store the staying solidified things in a protected refrigerator. Spot solidified ice packs or sacks of ice 3D shapes over the nourishment.

The nourishment will be protected to refreeze as long as it is still solidified strong.

To Freeze or Not?

egg whites), natural products, sauces, mix dishes, breads, cakes, and goulashes will all hold their quality very well in the cooler and will warm delightfully. Dealing with and readiness for capacity will be the key factors that decide if the nourishments will hold their quality when solidified and warmed.

Nourishments with a high water content (lettuce, tomatoes, radishes) don't stop well. All cells contain water, which extends when solidified. Cells of water-rich nourishments may separate a lot as the water inside them solidifies, bringing about an unsatisfactory taste or wet, soft surface when defrosted. Different nourishments that don't stop well include:

• Whole hard-cooked eggs

• Raw eggs

• Chopped or cut potatoes

• Celery

• Raw tomatoes

• Mayonnaise

• Custard and cream fillings

• Sour cream

• Fried nourishments

• Canned cooler mixture

It's conceivable to work around a portion of these issue nourishments. Buy effectively solidified things, for example, solidified potatoes; add them to the formula after it has cooled; at that point promptly solidify the dish. At the point when the formula is defrosted and warmed, the potatoes will be delicate and immaculate. Or on the other hand, you can likewise essentially let these nourishments well enough alone for the formula when you're setting it up for the cooler, at that point include them during the defrosting and warming procedure.

Rich dairy items can be solidified if a stabilizer is added to them, similar to flour or cornstarch. These things may isolate when defrosted, however, a basic blend with a wire whisk will smooth out the sauce.

Purchasing and Freezing Meat in Bulk

Meat falls into an exceptional class in once-a-month cooking. Since meat will be the most costly piece of your mass cooking buys, consistently search for deals on meat and include plans that utilization that meat to your arrangement. In any case, there are quite certain guidelines you have to pursue when acquiring and putting away enormous amounts of meat. Most significant, focus on lapse dates on meat items and never purchase or stop meat that is past those dates.

If you are obtaining huge amounts of meat previously solidified and plan to defrost the meat before utilizing it in plans, it must be cooked before being refrozen. Never defrost solidified meat, in part cook it or use it crudely in a formula, and refreeze it. Defrost solidified meat, at that point cook it totally, and it very well may be securely refrozen.

Try not to solidify meat in its unique bundling. Enclose it by cooler wrap, substantial foil, or zipper-lock cooler packs; name, and stop. Gap the meat into little amounts before you bundle it for refreezing so it will be simpler to defrost and work with. Stop chicken parts or fish filets independently, and afterward join in a bigger pack. Pork slashes ought to be isolated by cooler wrap, at that point joined in a bigger sack or wrapped together with cooler wrap. Enormous amounts of ground meat ought to be partitioned into meager bits and bundled separated by material or cooler paper.

Ensure you record the meats you are putting away in the cooler. When arranging each cooking session, allude to this rundown to utilize the meat put away in your cooler before you buy more. Most solidified meat will hold quality for a half year to a year. Restored meats like ham and bacon hold their quality in the cooler for just around one month. On account of the relieving procedure, these meats will, in general, oxidize quicker and will wind up rotten more rapidly than uncured meats.

Food Safety

Food safety is the most significant piece of any nourishment planning. It doesn't make a difference on the off chance that you get ready gourmet nourishments that everybody adores; if the nourishment makes individuals wiped out, all your work is lost. In the event that you have questions about the virtue or security of the nourishment, toss it out. These guidelines apply to all cooking and preparing, not simply once-a-month cooking.

Nourishments that could raise a ruckus whenever misused incorporate all crisp and restored meats (cooked and uncooked), eggs, dairy items like milk and cream, fish, cooked rice and pasta, opened or unlocked home-canned food sources, and all food sources that contain any of these fixings.

At whatever point you contact crude meats or uncooked eggs (even the shell!), promptly wash your hands with warm, sudsy water before contacting whatever else. Try not to open an organizer, get the salt shaker, or contact whatever will be eaten uncooked. Consider keeping a popup holder of hand wipes in your kitchen for comfort and to help you to remember this significant sanitation factor.

In excess of 75 million instances of food contamination happen in the United States each year. Practically all could be avoided by preparing nourishment to the best possible inside temperature. Pursue safe nourishment dealing with practices precisely.

Keep in mind, food contamination is undetectable—it is difficult to tell by taste or smell if nourishment is sheltered to eat. Most microbes and the poisons they produce, which cause nourishment borne ailments, are not distinguishable by human detects.

Nourishments ought to be left at room temperature for just two hours. By then, nourishments must be refrigerated or solidified. Microorganisms present in all nourishment develop at temperatures somewhere in the range of 40°F and 140°F. Ensure that you monitor to what extent possibly risky nourishment has been out of refrigeration.

For example, work with the majority of your ground meat plans—finish, cool, pack, mark, and stop them before going on to plans utilizing chicken. Keep crude meats separate from every other nourishment. Utilize a different cutting board, blade, and fork for getting ready crude meats. Regardless of whether the microscopic organisms in nourishment are killed in the cooking procedure, after some time, a few microbes produce poisons that are not devastated by warmth or frigid temperatures. Those poisons will make you wiped out. That is the reason you should pursue sanitation techniques exactly, warming nourishment rapidly, cooling it quickly, and never giving nourishment a chance to stand apart at room temperature for over two hours.

If somebody in your family falls into a high-chance gathering (has a traded off insusceptible framework or an incessant sickness, is older, or is younger than five), you should be significantly progressively cautious about sanitation. Individuals who fall into these high-hazard gatherings can become so ill structure food contamination they should be hospitalized.

PREPARING FOOD FOR THE FREEZER

The nourishment you go through throughout the day getting ready likewise must be appropriately stuffed, wrapped, and solidified to safeguard it in the most ideal quality. Also, before the nourishment can be pressed and solidified, it must be chilled.

Cool It!

Before putting the nourishment in your cooler, cool it as fast as possible. Hot nourishments will raise the temperature of your cooler and could bargain the wellbeing and nature of different nourishments put away there. At the point when the nourishment has been set up as the formula coordinates, place it in a metal cooking or heating container, in an ice-water shower, or spread the nourishment in a shallow skillet and spot it in the fridge for thirty to fifty minutes. At that point pack the nourishment in the cooler compartments or wrap, seal, mark, and stop right away.

Consider acquiring some enormous, strong, waterproof compartments or capacity containers to use as ice-water showers. You are going to require the majority of your blending bowls and pots for preparing the nourishment, and your sink will be brimming with sudsy water for cleaning.

Fast Freezing

This is essentially cold nourishments as fast as could be expected under the circumstances. Singular canapés, sandwiches, moves, treats, and other little size nourishments hold their quality, shape, and structure best when blaze solidified.

Spread a layer of nourishment on a treat sheet or another level surface and stop exclusively leave a space of one half to one inch between the individual bits of nourishment so cool air can circle uninhibitedly then bundle in one compartment once solidified strong.

Pack It!

Appropriate bundling and wrapping will keep your nourishment in incredible condition while it is being solidified and warmed. Ensure that there are no free wrappings around the nourishment. You can twofold wrap every formula after it has solidified strong to ensure that each bundle is appropriately fixed. Ensure you utilize rock-solid foil or cooler wrap that is heat-safe. Use cooler tape to seal creases when you use cooler wrap to bundle nourishment.

Try not to store tomato-based nourishments in foil; the corrosive in the tomatoes will eat through the foil, presenting the nourishment to air and gambling cooler consume. Utilize rock-solid heatproof cooler wrap for these nourishments.

The kinds of holders you use will decide how a lot of nourishment you'll have the option to store in your cooler. Block and flat bundles and holders utilize space, so you can include more bundles to the freezer Most goulashes can be solidified, expelled from their dishes, and after that stacked to store. To do this, line goulash and preparing dishes with rock-solid foil or cooler wrap. Amass the nourishment in the lined dishes, spread firmly with foil or cooler wrap, and stop. At the point when the nourishment is solidified strong, pop the nourishment out of the dish, wrap once more, and store. When you're prepared to eat, just spot the solidified nourishment over into the heating dish, defrost, and warm.

Load It!

Be certain the nourishment is altogether cooled before stacking your cooler. It's significant that nourishment that is

effectively solidified doesn't defrost or mollify in view of the expansion of unfrozen nourishment. Abstain from opening the cooler frequently during the stacking procedure. Rather, get together a few compartments and spot them in the cooler simultaneously. Each time you open the cooler, the temperature will rise a piece.

Consider separating your cooler into segments dependent on the plans it contains. Spot chicken plans in a single zone, hors d'oeuvres in a different bin or holder, and Slow Cooker plans in another region. You'll have the option to discover things all the more effectively, and you'll likewise have the option to see which formula class needs renewing when you're arranging your next once-a-month cooking session.

Forever append a note pad or dry eradicate load up to your cooler and update it each time you include or expel nourishment. Ensure that you've spent all the nourishment from your present cycle of once-a-month cooking before you plan another session.

Adding an excessive amount to your cooler without a moment's delay raises the temperature of the cooler and bargains the quality and wellbeing of your put away nourishment. Ensure that you never include what might be compared to in excess of 40 percent of your cooler space at once. Make certain to allude to the maker's guidance booklet for particulars for your sort and size of the freezer.

How to Thaw and Reheat

The second most important technique you need to learn to be a successful cooking and freezing expert is how to thaw and reheat foods. Some foods can be baked directly from the frozen state, while others come out better if thawed first. Each recipe in this book has complete thawing and reheating instructions. Follow these instructions carefully and use an instant-read thermometer to check the temperature of the food before serving.

Add thawing foods to your list of chores you do before bedtime, just as you choose your clothes

for the next day and check your children's homework. With a little extra planning, it's very simple to make a casserole from the freezer and store it in the refrigerator to thaw overnight, and then bake it the next evening.

When thawing meat in the refrigerator, place the bagged or wrapped meat in a container so the juices don't drip on any other food. Never thaw frozen meat at room temperature. You can thaw meat in the microwave oven, but only if you are going to cook it right away.

When you reheat thawed food, be sure it is fully cooked before serving it. Casseroles need to reach an internal temperature of 165°F before they are served. Test the casserole in the very center, since that is the last place to reach proper temperature. Meats must also be cooked to certain internal temperatures before they are safe to eat. Here are internal temperatures each meat type should reach when it is done.

ORGANIZING AND SELECTING RECIPES

Keep your cookbooks clean and in good condition by keeping them out of the kitchen. Copy recipes from this cookbook and your other favorites onto index cards. It's important to keep the recipes you use for freezing in a separate folder or notebook, along with any notes, lists, and changes to the recipes or lists that you have made. When you want to organize another cook-and-freeze session, all your information will be in one place. Clear vinyl page protectors will hold two 4" × 6" cards on each page in your recipe notebook.

Make photocopies of all of your recipes and tape them in easily accessible areas of your kitchen. You may want to tape recipes to cabinets or to the back of the kitchen door. This way, they stay out of the way, yet are always available when you need to refer to them.

Mix and Match

Think about serving one recipe in different ways. For instance, a beef chili recipe can be served

over taco chips and garnished with salsa, cheese, and lettuce as a taco salad. The same recipe can be served over baked potatoes or as a topping for hot dogs. This planning allows you to vary the meals you serve using your tried-and-true recipes, combining similar preparation and cooking steps.

When you are compiling your list of recipes, think not only about the foods your family likes, but also about what's on sale that week at your local supermarket. For instance, if your grocer has a special on ground beef in five-pound packs, pull recipes for meatloaf, spaghetti sauce, and beef

manicotti from your collection.

Variety Is Key

Make sure to choose a good variety of recipes for the month. For instance, choose several chicken casseroles, two grilled beef recipes, three slow cooker recipes, one chicken and one ham sandwich recipe, and a pepperoni pizza. Write down the recipes you have chosen on a blank calendar page; it's easier to make sure that you are serving your family a good variety of flavors, textures, colors, and nutrients during the month when you can see the whole month's plan at a glance.

What types of recipes should I choose from my own collection?

Simple recipes freeze best. Avoid recipes with complicated sauces, different cooking times, multiple preparation steps, and those that use exotic ingredients.

Cooking Day Dos and Don'ts

Since you're going to be spending the entire day cooking, the most important "do" of all is enjoy the process. Enjoy the sounds of cooking: the knife blade chunking into the chopping board, foods sizzling in a pan, and even the clink of metal on metal as you flip through nested measuring spoons.

Think about all the time you're going to save, and how well you are treating yourself and your family.

In addition:

Do stock up on paper towels and dishrags.

Do make sure you have several large plastic garbage bags available, and remove each bag from

the kitchen as soon as it is full.

Do cook with a helper or two. Split up some of the chores; for instance, one person can cook a

few recipes while the other keeps the kitchen clean, and then switch places.

Do keep a first-aid kit handy. When you're working with this much food and so many

appliances, it pays to be prepared.

Do make sure your knives are sharp and in good condition. A sharp knife slices more easily and

is actually safer to use than a dull knife. Dull knives can slip as you work with them, making it

all too easy to cut yourself.

Do make an inventory before you start, to make sure you have enough pots, pans, spoons, forks,

and knives on hand, and that they are all in good working order.

Do make sure that all your appliances are in good working order and are accurate.

Do schedule more time than you think you'll need.

Do take breaks where you leave the kitchen, sit down, and sip some tea while putting your feet

up. Nobody can work for seven or eight hours without a break.

Do think about prepping some of the food on the same day that you shop. You could cut up some

vegetables or meats and package them in plastic containers, or start meat cooking in your slow

cooker for the next day.

The most important "don't" of all: don't wear yourself out or undertake a day of cooking if you

don't feel well. If you're unsure of your strength or stamina, start small by choosing just a few meals to make and freeze. Here are some other important don'ts:

Don't attempt too much, especially on your first experience with this type of cooking. It's much

easier to schedule another cooking session if you aren't exhausted by the first attempt.

Don't shop and cook on the same day.

Don't let prepared food sit on the counter while you assemble other recipes. As soon as the

recipes are prepared, cool them, then pack, label, and freeze them.

Don't purchase frozen meats and then thaw and refreeze them without cooking. Once meat has

been thawed, it must be cooked before being refrozen.

Don't cook a meal for your family or yourself on C-day Go out to eat! You deserve some

pampering after your marathon cooking session.

Try to make your cooking session fun. If you see it as a positive challenge and do everything you

can to make the process enjoyable, you are going to want to schedule another session.

Load up your CD player with lots of songs you love. Upbeat songs with a good tempo will help

make the time fly. Makeup games as you go along. (Don't play timing games though; racing to see who can chop the most onions in a certain time frame, for instance, can only lead to disaster.)

Cook with a partner—a neighbor, relative, or work colleague. Think about organizing a cooking club and pair off with a different member each month. Your recipe collection will expand exponentially, and you'll pass along this efficient and money-saving cooking method to more people.

You will not only expand your collection of freezable recipes, but the time will go by much more

quickly when another person is there to share the chores. Enjoy the aromas as your home fills with delicious smells. Who needs potpourri or air fresheners when bread, cookies, casseroles, and vegetables are baking and simmering? And enjoy the safe, cozy feeling of "putting food by" to feed your family and friends.

CHAPTER 2

BULK COOKING MODEL

This chapter contains a complete one-month shopping and cooking plan. This plan will show you how to choose recipes; plan your shopping and "on-hand" lists; plan preparation of ingredients and cooking; prepare ingredients; assemble and cook recipes, and cool, wrap, and freeze the finished dishes.

Recipes for a Month

While you can certainly plan to cook thirty individual recipes for freezing, it's much easier to cook double or triple amounts of ten to fifteen recipes. When you think about it, your family usually requests the same recipe at least twice a month. You'll save lots of time and energy by doubling or tripling a recipe and packaging and freezing that food in meal-size portions. Then rotate the food into your meal plan for the month.

The ten recipes in this cooking model will be tripled, to make a total of thirty entrees that will

each serve four to six adults.

When choosing your recipes, you can make adjustments to streamline cooking. For instance, if one recipe calls for ground beef with onions and garlic and another uses just ground beef and onions, add garlic to the second dish or omit garlic from the first one so you can prepare the foods together.

It's important to make sure the recipes you have chosen are cooked with different methods. For

instance, you don't want to have thirty baked dishes unless you have three or four ovens. Choose some recipes that are cooked in a skillet or saucepan, some that are baked, some that are frozen without cooking, some that are grilled, and some that are prepared in a Slow Cooker.

Get Ready to Shop

Once you have collected your recipes, pull out a pencil and paper and start making your lists. Lists are your lifeline in this type of cooking. You'll need to create a shopping list and an "on-hand" list that will include every single ingredient listed in each recipe. You'll draw up these lists first, followed by a preparation schedule and a cooking schedule.

Make copies of your recipes to make it easier to work on these lists. Then, using the Equivalents

Chart (Commonly Used Cooking Equivalents), convert cups into pounds and ounces, and convert can and bottle sizes. Go through each recipe, writing down each ingredient on your on-hand list if you have it or on the shopping list if you don't, and check off each ingredient as you go. Double-check your lists; your cooking session will be a disaster if you are missing ingredients. You might want to practice making your own shopping and on-hand lists from this session's recipes, then compare them to the lists that follow. (Your own shopping and on-hand lists may be slightly different, depending on what's in your pantry and freezer, and the substitutions you use for the recipes.)

The following are the shopping and on-hand lists for the above recipes.

Be sure to double-check your lists and make sure all ingredients, preparation steps, and cooking

steps are included.

Make notes as you go through preparation and cooking, to improve your assembly-line process, refine shopping lists and organization of tools and ingredients, and streamline recipe preparation.

Shortcuts

Depending on your schedule and pocketbook, there are lots of shortcuts available for this cooking plan. If you aren't watching sodium or fat content in your diet, purchasing sauces, gravies, mixes, and other prepared ingredients can save a lot of time. Other shortcuts you might be interested in include the following:

• Purchase canned or bottled chicken gravy for Chicken on Cornbread and Chicken Pot Pie.

• Use a corn muffin mix to make the cornbread.

• Use frozen or refrigerated pie crusts instead of making them from scratch.

• Buy pre-cooked chicken that is sliced or cubed, either from the deli or the frozen foods section of the supermarket.

• Buy precooked, preseasoned ground beef from the meat section of the supermarket.

• Purchase grated and shredded cheese from the deli or dairy section of the supermarket.

• Buy prepared vegetables from a salad bar in your supermarket.

• Purchase cooked rice from a local Chinese restaurant.

• Buy coleslaw mix instead of shredding cabbage; purchase one head of cabbage for the recipe that requires whole leaves.

• Purchase 6 pounds of meatloaf mix instead of 3 each of ground beef and ground pork.

Remember, these shortcuts will cost more than buying items that aren't "value-added." Decide whether your budget can handle these added conveniences and whether the time you will save is worth the extra cost.

Planning and Preparation

There are some tasks that you can do ahead of the cooking day. Place all non-perishable foods on your kitchen table in groups as they are needed for the recipes to make sure you have all the ingredients on hand. This can be done two to three days ahead of cooking day. The following preparation steps can be done either the day before or on the morning of cooking day itself.

• Cook the 12 pounds of bone-in chicken breasts in your slow cooker in batches of 4 pounds each for 6 to 7 hours on low, simmer in water for 30 to 45 minutes, or bake in the oven for 50 to 60 minutes. Refrigerate, covered, until needed. (If you cook your chicken by simmering, reserve the broth and use it in place of purchased condensed chicken broth.)

• Peel and chop the onions and garlic, place in zipper-lock bags, and store in the refrigerator.

• Seed and chop the red bell peppers, place in zipper-lock bags, and store in the refrigerator.

• Make pie crust dough, roll out between sheets of waxed paper, wrap again, and refrigerate.

• Cook wild rice until almost tender; drain and refrigerate.

Time for a break! Make yourself a cup of coffee and sit in a comfortable chair while the wild rice

is cooking. Put your feet up on an ottoman and listen to some music. Do some simple stretching

exercises or massage your feet.

• Seed and chop the jalapenos and green chilies and store in zipper-lock bags in the refrigerator.

• Grate carrots and store in zipper-lock bags in the refrigerator.

• Remove 24 leaves of cabbage from heads; core heads and shred remaining cabbage. Store in zipper-lock bags in the refrigerator.

• Shred the cheeses and store in zipper-lock bags in the refrigerator.

• Group all of the non-perishable and canned foods that you need for each recipe together.

• Divide chicken thighs and boneless chicken breasts into three equal portions each, package in zipper-lock bags, label, and freeze for Slow Cooker Spicy Peanut Chicken and Italian Slow Cooker Chicken.

Time to Get Cooking!

Now that the shopping and preparation phases are complete, it's time to start some serious cooking.

As you finish each dish, place it in the refrigerator or in an ice bath to cool quickly, or freeze immediately, depending on the recipe. When the food is cold, fold wrapping over the food, seal seams, overwrap if necessary, label, and place it in the freezer. Be sure to carefully seal all seams in freezer paper using freezer tape.

Label foods accurately as you go along. Once meals are wrapped and frozen, it will be difficult to identify them. Waterproof markers, grease pencils, and wax markers work well on most freezer wrap and plastic containers. Be sure to record the name of the recipe, the date it was prepared, thawing and reheating instructions, and additional foods needed to finish the recipe.

When casseroles are frozen solid, you can remove them from the baking dishes, then wrap again in freezer wrap or foil and stack to save room. Make sure to rotate food as you add it to your freezer, placing the items frozen for the longest time on top or in the front of the freezer so you'll use them first.

The following steps will see you through the rest of your cooking day:

• If you haven't already cooked the chicken, bake the 12 pounds of bone-in chicken breasts.

Sprinkle chicken with salt and pepper and place in several large pans. Cover with foil and bake at 350°F for 30 minutes. Uncover and bake 20 to 30 minutes longer or until meat thermometer registers 170°F. When chicken is done, remove from oven and place in refrigerator until cool enough to handle. Or cook chicken by placing in a stockpot, cover with water, and simmering for 30 to 45 minutes until done. Reserve the broth for your recipes.

• Wash and chop the mushrooms, and prepare any other vegetables you didn't prepare the day before.

• Start cooking the wild rice (if you didn't already) and the white rice and mix the cornbread batter.

Bake cornbread until set. When rice is cooked until almost tender, drain if necessary and set aside.

• Combine the recipes for the gravy for Chicken Pot Pie and Chicken on Cornbread in a large stockpot. Let simmer for 5 to 6 minutes. Then chill in the refrigerator.

• Remove meat from cooked and cooled chicken; freeze skin and bones to make broth later if desired. Slice half of chicken and cube half; store in the refrigerator.

• Assemble sauce for Slow Cooker Spicy Peanut Chicken and pour into containers. Attach to bag of chicken thighs, label, and freeze. Set aside couscous in pantry, marked as "reserved."

Time for a break! Do some simple stretches and breathe deeply. Think about changing your shoes to rest your feet. Have a snack of some fresh fruit and cold water or iced tea.

• Add sliced chicken to half of chicken gravy for Chicken on Cornbread. Wrap cornbread, attach bag of chicken in gravy, label, and freeze.

• Combine sauce ingredients for Italian Slow Cooker Chicken and pour into three one-quart zipper-lock bags. Attach three zipper-lock bags of boneless chicken breasts and three more bags with potatoes, label, and freeze.

• Sauté 3 cups chopped onions and 3 cloves minced garlic in olive oil for Wild Rice Meatloaf; refrigerate.

• Sauté, in batches, 9 pounds ground beef, 9 onions, and 27 cloves garlic, minced, for Easy Lasagna, Cabbage Rolls, and Spaghetti. Drain and refrigerate as the meat is cooked; divide mixture into three equal portions. Add pasta sauce and water to one portion for Easy Lasagna and set aside in the fridge.

• Combine all ingredients for Wild Rice Meatloaf and shape it into three loaves. Bake as directed until done, then refrigerate until cold.

• Mix lasagna cheese filling; then assemble lasagnas in three-lined pans; refrigerate.

• Add thyme, red bell pepper, chicken, and frozen vegetables to chilled chicken gravy for Chicken

CHAPTER THREE

COOKING RECIPES

Cheesy Tomato Gougere Puffs

To serve immediately, bake puffs at 375ºF for 75 to 20 minutes or until puffed and browned. Remove from oven and cut a tiny slit in each puff to let out steam.

Makes 48

1 cup milk

¼ cup butter

½ teaspoon salt

Pinch white pepper

1 cup flour

4 eggs

¼ cup oil-packed sun-dried tomatoes

1 cup crumbled blue cheese

1 egg yolk

2 teaspoons water

¼ cup grated Parmesan cheese

Makes 144

3 cups of milk

¾ cup butter

1½ teaspoons salt

teaspoon white pepper

3 cups flour

12 eggs

¾ cup oil-packed sun-dried tomatoes

3 cups crumbled blue cheese

3 egg yolks

6 teaspoons water

¾ cup grated Parmesan cheese

1. Preheat oven to 375°F. In heavy saucepan, combine milk, butter, salt, and white pepper and bring to a rolling boil. Add flour all at once, stirring constantly. Cook over medium heat, stirring constantly, until ball of dough forms and cleans sides of pan.

2. Using electric mixer, beat in eggs, one at a time. Remove from heat and let cool for 20 minutes.

Drain sun-dried tomatoes well, then mince. Add tomatoes and blue cheese to dough. Stir to combine.

3. Drop teaspoons of dough onto baking sheets lined with parchment paper. Beat egg yolk and water in small bowl and carefully brush over each puff. Sprinkle with Parmesan cheese. Bake at 375°F for 15 to 20 minutes or until puffed, golden brown, and firm. Flash freeze puffs on baking sheet; and then pack, wrap, label, and freeze.

4. To reheat: Bake frozen puffs at 375°F for 4 to 6 minutes or until hot.

Seafood Turnovers

To serve immediately, bake at 400°F for 18 to 23 minutes or until pastry is golden brown and filling is hot.

Makes 24

1 (6-ounce) can small shrimp, drained

½ cup ricotta cheese

3 green onions, finely chopped

1 cup shredded Havarti cheese

½ teaspoon dried dill weed

1 sheet frozen puff pastry, thawed

1 egg yolk, beaten

1 tablespoon water

Makes 72

3 (6-ounce) cans small shrimp, drained

1½ cups ricotta cheese

9 green onions, finely chopped

3 cups shredded Havarti cheese

1½ teaspoons dried dill weed

3 sheets frozen puff pastry, thawed

3 egg yolks, beaten

3 tablespoons water

1. In medium bowl, combine shrimp, ricotta, green onions, Havarti, and dill weed and mix well.

2. Gently roll puff pastry into 12-inch by 18-inch rectangle. Cut into 24 3-inch squares. Place 2 teaspoons shrimp mixture in center of each square. Beat egg yolk with water in small bowl.

Brush edges of pastry with egg yolk mixture. Fold puff pastry over filling, forming triangles; press edges with fork to seal.

3. Flash freeze turnovers in a single layer on the baking sheet. Then pack in rigid containers, with waxed paper separating the layers. Label containers and freeze.

4. To reheat: Preheat oven to 450°F. Place frozen turnovers on a baking sheet. Bake at 450°F for 4 minutes; then turn oven down to 400°F and bake for 12 to 15 minutes longer or until pastry is golden and filling is hot.

Sticky Roast Chicken

To serve this delicious dish without freezing, marinate chicken for 4 to 8 hours in the refrigerator, then roast the chicken as directed.

Serves 4–6

4 pounds chicken, cut into serving pieces

1 cup honey

1 teaspoon salt

3 tablespoons balsamic

vinegar

2 tablespoons olive oil

1 teaspoon paprika

1 teaspoon pepper

½ teaspoon cayenne pepper

3 cloves garlic, minced

Serves 12–18

12 pounds chicken, cut into serving pieces

1 cup honey

1 tablespoon salt

9 tablespoons balsamic vinegar

6 tablespoons olive oil

1 tablespoon paprika

1 teaspoon pepper

1½ teaspoons cayenne pepper

9 cloves garlic, minced

1. Place chicken pieces in a 1-gallon zipper-lock bag. In medium bowl, mix remaining ingredients and pour over chicken. Seal bag, label, and freeze.

2. To thaw and cook: Thaw chicken and sauce overnight in refrigerator. Preheat oven to 325°F.

Place chicken pieces and sauce in 9″ × 13″ baking pan; roast at 325°F for 60 to 75 minutes until instant-read thermometer reads 180°F To make a sauce from the pan drippings, place pan over medium heat and add ½ cup chicken broth; bring to a boil.

Pesto Drumsticks

To serve these tender and juicy drumsticks immediately, bake as directed without freezing. Serve with mashed potatoes and cooked peas drizzled with a little melted butter.

Serves 4–6

8 chicken drumsticks

½ teaspoon salt

1 teaspoon pepper

¼ cup Pesto Sauce

½ cup Chicken Broth

2 tablespoons lemon juice

Serves 12–18

24 chicken drumsticks

1½ teaspoons salt

¼ teaspoon pepper

¾ cup Pesto Sauce

1½ cups Chicken Broth

6 tablespoons lemon juice

1. Sprinkle drumsticks with salt and pepper. Carefully loosen the skin of drumsticks and spread pesto over flesh. Smooth skin back into place. In small bowl, combine chicken broth and lemon juice. Place drumsticks in zipper-lock bags and pour chicken broth and lemon juice over. Label and freeze.

2. To thaw and reheat: Thaw drumsticks overnight in refrigerator. Place drumsticks and sauce in 13″ × 9″ baking dish. Cover and bake

at 350°F for 30 minutes. Uncover casserole and baste drumsticks with liquid in pan. Bake, uncovered, for 20 to 30 minutes longer, until chicken is thoroughly cooked (meat thermometer registers 180°F).

Cannellini Chicken Soup

This hearty soup can be served without freezing by simmering for 40 to 45 minutes, then add drained and rinsed cannellini beans. Simmer soup for another 10 to 15 minutes, until slightly thickened.

Serves 4

1 pound boned, skinned chicken thighs

1 onion, chopped

3 cloves garlic, minced

3 tablespoons olive oil

1 tablespoon butter

3 carrots, sliced

4 cups Chicken Broth

1 teaspoon salt

1 teaspoon white pepper

½ teaspoon dried marjoram leaves

2 (16-ounce) cans cannellini beans

½ cup grated Parmesan cheese

Serves 12

3 pounds boned, skinned chicken thighs

3 onions, chopped

9 cloves garlic, minced

9 tablespoons olive oil

3 tablespoons butter

9 carrots, sliced

12 cups Chicken Broth

1 tablespoon salt

1 teaspoon white pepper

1½ teaspoons dried marjoram leaves

6 (16-ounce) cans cannellini beans

1½ cups grated Parmesan cheese

1. Cut chicken into 1-inch pieces. Sauté chicken, onion, and garlic in olive oil and butter in large

stockpot until chicken is browned and vegetables are crisp-tender. Add carrots; cook and stir 4 to 5 minutes. Add broth, salt, pepper, and marjoram and bring to a boil. Reduce heat, cover, and simmer for 30 to 35 minutes, until chicken is thoroughly cooked.

2. Chill soup in an ice-water bath or refrigerator. Drain and rinse beans and add to chilled soup. Pour soup into a 1-gallon zipper-lock bag and attach a small bag with Parmesan cheese. Label and freeze.

3. To thaw and reheat: Tet soup thaw overnight in refrigerator. Pour into heavy saucepan or stockpot and simmer for 10 to 15 minutes, until thoroughly heated. Serve topped with Parmesan cheese.

White and Green Lasagna

This easy lasagna doesn't use any tomato products. To serve immediately sprinkle cheese on the casserole and bake at 375°F for 20 to 30 minutes, until bubbly and cheese begins to brown.

Serves 6

3 tablespoons olive oil

2 tablespoons butter

1 onion, chopped

¼ cup flour

½ cup Chicken Broth

1 cup milk

1 cup shredded Monterey jack cheese

½ cup grated Romano cheese

3 cups cooked, cubed chicken

1 (9-ounce) package frozen cut-leaf spinach

2 cups ricotta cheese

1 egg

1 cup grated Parmesan cheese

1 (4-ounce) jar sliced mushrooms, drained

9 lasagna noodles

1 cup grated Parmesan cheese

Serves 18

9 tablespoons olive oil

6 tablespoons butter

3 onions, chopped

¾ cup flour

1½ cups Chicken Broth

3 cups of milk

3 cups shredded Monterey jack cheese

1½ cups grated Romano cheese

9 cups cooked, cubed chicken

3 (9 ounce) packages frozen

1 cut leaf spinach

6 cups ricotta cheese

3 eggs

3 cups grated Parmesan cheese

3 (4 ounce) jars sliced mushrooms, drained

27 lasagna noodles

3 cups grated Parmesan cheese

1. In a large skillet, heat olive oil and butter. Add onion; cook and stir until crisp-tender, about 4 to 5 minutes. Sprinkle flour over onion; cook and stir until bubbly. Add broth and milk; cook and stir until thickened and bubbly. Add Monterey Jack cheese, Romano cheese, and cubed chicken. Mix well and set aside.

2. Thaw spinach and drain by pressing between paper towels. In large bowl, combine ricotta cheese, egg, first quantity Parmesan cheese, drained spinach, and mushrooms. Cook lasagna noodles until almost done, according to package directions. Drain well and rinse with cold water.

3. In 13″ × 9″ baking dish, place ½ cup chicken sauce. Top with three lasagna noodles, then with half of spinach mixture. Then top with more chicken sauce. Repeat layers, ending with chicken sauce. Chill in an ice-water bath or in refrigerator, wrap, label, and attach small bag with 1 cup grated Parmesan cheese; then freeze.

4. To thaw and reheat: Thaw overnight in refrigerator. Preheat oven to 375°. Sprinkle lasagna with Parmesan cheese. Bake at 375°F for 30 to 40 minutes, until casserole is hot in center, cheese is brown, and sauce bubbles.

Spicy Chicken Pizza

Prebaking the pizza crust makes it stay crisp through freezing and reheating. To serve immediately, bake the pizza as soon as it is assembled at 400°F for 15 to 20 minutes.

Serves 6

1 12-inch round Pizza Crust

1 (8-ounce) can tomato sauce

3 tablespoons tomato paste

¼ teaspoon crushed red pepper flakes

2 cups cooked, cubed chicken

1 cup frozen onions and peppers

½ cup ricotta cheese

2 cups shredded Colby-jack cheese

½ cup grated Parmesan cheese

Serves 18

3 12-inch round Pizza Crusts

3 (8-ounce) cans tomato sauce

9 tablespoons tomato paste

¾ teaspoon crushed red pepper flakes

6 cups cooked, cubed chicken

3 cups frozen onions and peppers

1½ cups ricotta cheese

6 cups shredded Colby-jack cheese

1½ cups grated Parmesan cheese

1. Preheat oven to 400°F. Prebake pizza crust at 400°F for 10 minutes, until set. Cool on wire rack. In small bowl, combine tomato sauce, tomato paste, and crushed red pepper flakes; spread over cooled crust.

2. Top pizza with chicken and frozen onions and peppers. Drop ricotta cheese by small spoonfuls over chicken. Top with Colby-jack and Parmesan; flash freeze on a baking sheet. Wrap frozen pizza in freezer wrap; seal, label, and freeze.

3. To reheat: Take frozen pizza in preheated 400°F oven for 18 to 25 minutes, until thoroughly heated and cheese is melted and bubbly.

Creamy Peanut Chicken

To serve without freezing, cook chicken and onion mixture in olive oil for 7 to 8 minutes. Add sauce and simmer for another 10 to 15 minutes, until chicken is thoroughly cooked.

Serves 4–6

2 pounds boned, skinned chicken thighs

1 onion, chopped

2 tablespoons olive oil

2 cups Chicken Broth

½ cup peanut butter

2 tablespoons soy sauce

½ cup evaporated milk

½ teaspoon salt

1 teaspoon pepper

2 tablespoons lemon juice

2 tablespoons honey

½ cup chopped peanuts

Serves 12–18

6 pounds boned, skinned chicken thighs

3 onions, chopped

6 tablespoons olive oil

6 cups Chicken Broth

1½ cups peanut butter

6 tablespoons soy sauce

1½ cups evaporated milk

1½ teaspoons salt

1 teaspoon pepper

6 tablespoons lemon juice

6 tablespoons honey

1½ cups chopped peanuts

1. Freeze chicken for 1 hour so it's easier to slice. Then cut chicken into 1-inch strips and refrigerate. In heavy skillet, sauté onion in olive oil until crisp-tender. Cool in refrigerator.

When cool, place chicken strips and sautéed onion in zipper-lock bags and place in the freezer.

2. In medium bowl, combine chicken broth, peanut butter, soy sauce, evaporated milk, salt, pepper, lemon juice, and honey and mix well to blend. Pour into another zipper-lock bag and attach it to chicken along with a small bag of chopped peanuts. Label bags and freeze.

3. To thaw and reheat: Thaw all bags overnight in refrigerator. Heat 2 tablespoons olive oil in heavy skillet. Add chicken mixture and cook, stirring frequently, for 7 to 8 minutes. Add sauce mixture and bring to a boil. Simmer chicken and sauce for 10 to 20 minutes, until chicken is thoroughly cooked, stirring frequently. Sprinkle dish with chopped peanuts and serve.

Chicken Pot Pie

To serve this recipe without freezing, heat chicken and vegetables in gravy until bubbly. Pour into 10-inch deep-dish pie pan. Place pastry on top, flute, and cut decorative holes. Bake at 400°F for 30 to 35 minutes, until crust is golden brown and filling is bubbly.

Serves 4–6

¼ cup butter

¼ cup minced onion

¼ cup flour

½ teaspoon salt

1 teaspoon pepper

1 cup Chicken Broth

½ cup milk

½ teaspoon dried thyme leaves

2 cups cooked, cubed chicken

1 cup chopped red bell pepper

2 cups frozen peas and carrots

1 cup frozen Southern-style hash brown potatoes

1 Pie Crust

Serves 12–18

¾ cup butter

¾ cup minced onion

¾ cup flour

1 teaspoon salt

1 teaspoon pepper

3 cups Chicken Broth

1½ cups milk

1½ teaspoons dried thyme leaves

6 cups cooked, cubed chicken

3 cups chopped red bell pepper

6 cups frozen peas and carrots

3 cups frozen Southern-style hash brown potatoes

3 Pie Crusts

1. Preheat oven to 400°F. In large saucepan, melt butter; add onion, cook and stir over medium heat until crisp-tender, about 4 to 5 minutes. Add flour, salt, and pepper to saucepan. Cook and stir until bubbly, about 3 to 4 minutes. Add broth and milk and stir; cook 5 to 6 minutes, until mixture is thickened and bubbly.

2. Add thyme, chicken, and bell pepper to mixture in saucepan. Cool mixture in refrigerator until cold, and then stir in frozen vegetables and frozen potatoes. Pour gravy with chicken and vegetables into deep-dish 10-inch pie pan.

3. Roll out pastry between pieces of waxed paper into a 10-inch circle. Cover pie with pastry round, crimp edges, and cut vent holes. Wrap pie, label, and freeze.

4. To thaw and reheat: Thaw pie overnight in refrigerator. Remove wrapping and bake at 400°F for 65 to 85 minutes, or until filling is bubbling in center and crust is golden brown. Let stand 10 minutes before serving.

Roasted Turkey Breast

To serve immediately, roast turkey breast as directed below. Remove from oven, cover, and let stand 10 minutes before carving. Serve with pan juices.

Serves 8–10

1 (5-pound) turkey breast

2 teaspoons seasoned salt

1 teaspoon white pepper

1 teaspoon dried marjoram leaves

1 teaspoon dried thyme leaves

2 tablespoons butter, melted

2 tablespoons olive oil

1 cup Chicken Broth

Serves 24–30

3 (5-pound) turkey breasts

6 teaspoons seasoned salt

1 teaspoon white pepper

1 tablespoon dried marjoram leaves

1 tablespoon dried thyme leaves

6 tablespoons butter, melted

6 tablespoons olive oil

3 cups Chicken Broth

1. Preheat oven to 325°F. Loosen skin from turkey breast, being careful not to tear skin. In small bowl, combine salt, pepper,

marjoram, thyme, butter, and olive oil and mix well. Spread this mixture over the turkey flesh. Smooth skin back over turkey.

2. Place turkey on rack in baking pan and pour chicken broth overall. Roast at 325°F for 2½ to 3 hours, until internal temperature registers 180°F, basting occasionally with pan juices.

3. Cool turkey and juices in the refrigerator until cold. Sliced turkey (leaving skin on slices if desired) and place it in a zipper-lock bag. Pour juices over, seal bag, label, and freeze.

4. To thaw and reheat: Thaw overnight in refrigerator. Place turkey slices and juices in heavy skillet. Heat turkey over medium heat for 8 to 12 minutes, shaking pan occasionally, until slices are thoroughly heated and juices boil.

Turkey Cassoulet

To serve immediately, pour turkey mixture into the baking dish after simmering and bake at 375°F for 15 minutes. Sprinkle with bread crumb mixture and bake 75 minutes longer.

Serves 8–10

2 pounds boneless, skinless turkey breast

4 slices bacon, chopped

3 tablespoons olive oil

2 onions, chopped

4 cloves garlic, chopped

1 cup Chicken Broth

2 (16-ounce) cans cannellini beans, drained

3 carrots, sliced

2 (14-ounce) cans diced tomatoes, undrained

1 teaspoon dried thyme leaves

1 teaspoon dried marjoram leaves

1 teaspoon pepper

1 cup whole wheat bread crumbs

2 tablespoons olive oil

¼ cup grated Parmesan cheese

Serves 24–30

6 pounds boneless, skinless turkey breast

12 slices bacon, chopped

9 tablespoons olive oil

6 onions, chopped

12 cloves garlic, chopped

3 cups Chicken Broth

6 (16-ounce) cans cannellini beans, drained

9 carrots, sliced

6 (14-ounce) cans diced tomatoes, undrained

1 tablespoon dried thyme leaves

1 tablespoon dried marjoram leaves

1 teaspoon pepper

3 cups whole wheat bread crumbs

6 tablespoons olive oil

¾ cup grated Parmesan cheese

1. Cut turkey into 1½-inch pieces. In large stockpot, cook bacon until crisp. Remove from pan and drain on paper towels. Add first quantity of olive oil to pan and cook turkey in batches, until the cubes begin to brown. Remove from pan as they are browned.

2. Add onion and garlic to pan and cook and stir until crisp-tender. Deglaze pan by pouring in broth and scraping up drippings; then add remaining ingredients except for bread crumbs, 2 tablespoons olive oil, and Parmesan cheese. Cover pan and simmer for 20 to 25 minutes or until turkey is thoroughly cooked and vegetables are tender.

3. Cool cassoulet in ice-water bath or in refrigerator. When cold, package in rigid containers. Combine bread crumbs, olive oil, and cheese and place in a small zipper-lock bag. Attach to cassoulet, label, and freeze.

4. To thaw and reheat: Thaw overnight in refrigerator. Preheat oven to 375°F. Place turkey mixture in a 2-quart baking dish. Cover and bake at 375°F for 30 to 40 minutes or until bubbly.

Uncover, sprinkle bread crumb mixture over, and bake 10 to 15 minutes longer, until topping is

crisp.

Orange Glazed Turkey Cutlets

Turkey cutlets are also known as turkey tenders. To serve immediately simmer cutlets in sauce for 5 to 10 minutes, and serve over hot cooked rice or egg noodles.

Serves 6–8

2 pounds turkey cutlets

1 teaspoon salt

1 teaspoon white pepper

2 tablespoons olive oil

2 tablespoons butter

1 cup of orange juice

1 tablespoon Worcestershire sauce

2 tablespoons honey

1 teaspoon dried basil leaves

1 tablespoon white wine vinegar

Serves 18–24

6 pounds turkey cutlets

1 tablespoon salt

1 teaspoon white pepper

6 tablespoons olive oil

6 tablespoons butter

3 cups orange juice

3 tablespoons Worcestershire sauce

6 tablespoons honey 1 tablespoon dried basil leaves

3 tablespoons white wine vinegar

1. Sprinkle cutlets with salt and white pepper. Heat olive oil and butter in large skillet over medium heat until foamy. Add cutlets and cook in batches, turning once, for 3 to 4 minutes per side, until turkey is thoroughly cooked. Remove cutlets as they cook.

2. To make sauce, add remaining ingredients to the pan. Cook and stir over medium heat until bubbly. Chill turkey and sauce in an ice-water bath or refrigerator. Pack into zipper-lock bags, label, and freeze.

3. To thaw and reheat: Thaw in refrigerator overnight. Place turkey and sauce in heavy skillet. Cook over medium heat, stirring occasionally, about 8 to 9 minutes or until cutlets are hot and sauce bubbles.

Turkey Meatloaf

This tender loaf is full of flavor. To serve without freezing, let fully cooked meatloaf stand, covered, 10 minutes before slicing.

Serves 6

1 onion, chopped

2 cups mushrooms, finely chopped

3 cloves garlic, minced

2 tablespoons olive oil

½ cup dry bread crumbs

¼ cup evaporated milk

1 egg

1 teaspoon salt

1 teaspoon white pepper

½ teaspoon dried marjoram leaves

2 pounds ground turkey

Serves 18

3 onions, chopped

6 cups mushrooms, finely chopped

9 cloves garlic, minced

6 tablespoons olive oil

1½ cups dry bread crumbs

¾ cup evaporated milk

3 eggs

1 tablespoon salt

1 teaspoon white pepper

1½ teaspoons dried marjoram leaves

6 pounds ground turkey

1. Preheat oven to 350°F. In heavy skillet, cook onions, mushrooms, and garlic in olive oil until vegetables are tender. Remove from heat and set aside.

2. In large bowl, combine bread crumbs, milk, egg, salt, pepper, and marjoram and mix well. Add sautéed vegetable mixture and stir to blend. Add ground turkey and mix gently with hands. Form mixture into oblong loaf and place on baking pan. Bake at 350°F for 50 to 60 minutes, until instant-read thermometer measures 170°F Cool meatloaf in the refrigerator; then wrap, label, and freeze.

3. To thaw and reheat: Thaw meatloaf overnight in refrigerator. It can be served cold at this point, or to reheat, place meatloaf on baking pan and brush with chicken broth. Bake at 350°F for 20 to 35 minutes, until thoroughly heated.

Curried Turkey Casserole

To serve without freezing, when casserole is assembled, bake at 375°F for 20 to 30 minutes, until thoroughly heated.

Serves 4–6

2 turkey tenderloins

1 tablespoon curry powder

¼ cup flour

1 teaspoon salt

2 tablespoons olive oil

1½ cups apple juice

1 tablespoon grated gingerroot

½ cup sour cream

2 cups Chicken Broth

1 teaspoon saffron

1 cup long-grain rice

3 carrots, sliced

Serves 12–18

6 turkey tenderloins

3 tablespoons curry powder

¾ cup flour

1 tablespoon salt

6 tablespoons olive oil

4½ cups apple juice

3 tablespoons grated ginger root

1½ cups sour cream

6 cups Chicken Broth

1 teaspoon saffron

3 cups long-grain rice

9 carrots, sliced

1. Cut turkey into 1-inch cubes. On shallow plate, combine curry powder, flour, and salt and mix well. Add turkey cubes and toss to coat well. Heat olive oil in heavy skillet and add coated turkey in batches. Cook and stir turkey until browned, about 4 to 5 minutes. Add apple juice and gingerroot to turkey and simmer 20 minutes. Add sour cream and remove from heat.

2. In saucepan, bring chicken broth and saffron to a boil. Add rice, cover, reduce heat, and simmer for 15 minutes or until almost tender. Add rice to turkey mixture; then add carrots. Place in 2-quart casserole dish, wrap, seal, label, and freeze.

3. To thaw and reheat: Thaw casserole overnight in refrigerator. Bake in preheated 375°F oven for 30 to 35 minutes or until thoroughly heated.

Glazed Turkey Breast

To serve without freezing, roast turkey as directed. When internal temperature reaches 180°F, let turkey stand, covered, for 10 minutes before slicing. Serve with cooked rice.

Serves 6–8

1 (5-pound) boneless turkey breast

1 teaspoon salt teaspoon white pepper

1 cup honey

1 cup of orange juice

3 tablespoons lime juice

2 teaspoons dried basil

Serves 18–24

3 (5-pound) boneless turkey breasts

1 tablespoon salt

1 teaspoon white pepper

1 cup honey

3 cups orange juice

9 tablespoons lime juice

2 tablespoons dried basil

1. Preheat oven to 325°F. Loosen skin from turkey breast. In small bowl, combine all remaining ingredients. Brush some of this mixture on the flesh under the skin. Gently smooth skin back into place and brush the entire turkey breast with this mixture.

2. Coat roasting pan with nonstick cooking spray. Place breast in roasting pan, skin-side down, and pour half of sauce over. Roast at

325°F for 1 hour. Turn turkey over and cover with remaining sauce. Continue roasting for 60 to 90 minutes, basting occasionally with pan juices, until turkey registers 180°F on an instant-read thermometer. Cool turkey in refrigerator and slice. Place slices in zipper-lock bags and pour pan juices over turkey; freeze.

3. To thaw and reheat: Thaw overnight in refrigerator. Place turkey slices and pan juices in heavy skillet. Heat turkey over medium heat for 8 to 12 minutes, shaking pan occasionally, until slices are thoroughly heated and juices boil.

Turkey Pot Pie

To serve without freezing, do not cool sauce. Add cheese, turkey, and vegetables and pour into pie pan. Add pastry and bake as directed.

Serves 6–8

1 onion, chopped

1 leek, chopped

2 tablespoons butter

2 tablespoons olive oil

¼ cup flour

1 teaspoon salt

1 teaspoon pepper

1 teaspoon dried thyme leaves

1 cup Chicken Broth

1 cup evaporated milk

½ cup grated Parmesan cheese

2 cups cubed, cooked turkey

1 cup frozen mixed vegetables

1 sheet frozen puff pastry

1 egg

Serves 18–24

3 onions, chopped

3 leeks, chopped

6 tablespoons butter

6 tablespoons olive oil

¾ cup flour

1 tablespoon salt

1 teaspoon pepper

1 tablespoon dried thyme leaves

3 cups Chicken Broth

3 cups evaporated milk

1½ cups grated Parmesan cheese

6 cups cubed, cooked turkey

3 cups frozen mixed vegetables

3 sheets frozen puff pastry

3 eggs

1. In heavy skillet, sauté onion and leek in butter and olive oil over medium heat until crisp-tender. Sprinkle with flour, salt, pepper, and thyme. Cook and stir until mixture bubbles, 3 to 4 minutes.

Add broth and evaporated milk; cook and stir until sauce thickens. Remove from heat and stir in

Parmesan cheese.

2. Cool sauce in an ice-water bath or refrigerator. Stir in cooked turkey and frozen vegetables. Pour into lined 9-inch deep-dish pie pan, wrap, seal, and attach wrapped puff pastry; freeze. Reserve egg in refrigerator.

3. To thaw and reheat: Thaw pie and pastry overnight in refrigerator. Preheat oven to 400°F. Cut a 10-inch circle from puff pastry and place over turkey mixture in pie plate. Seal edges, brush with beaten egg, and bake pie at 400°F for 50 to 60 minutes, until filling bubbles in center and crust is golden brown.

Turkey Tenderloins with Blueberry Compote

Tender turkey slices are deliciously contrasted with cold spicy-fruity compote. To serve immediately marinate turkey in refrigerator for 2 hours; cook as directed.

Serves 6

1 teaspoon salt

1 teaspoon white pepper

1 tablespoon white wine vinegar

1 tablespoon honey

1 tablespoon olive oil

2 turkey tenderloins

2 cups frozen blueberries

¼ cup minced onion

2 cloves garlic, minced

¼ cup orange juice

¼ teaspoons cinnamon

2 tablespoons sugar

Serves 18

1 tablespoon salt

1 teaspoon white pepper

3 tablespoons white wine vinegar

3 tablespoons honey

3 tablespoons plus 2 tablespoons olive oil

6 turkey tenderloins

6 cups frozen blueberries

¾ cup minced onion

6 cloves garlic, minced

¾ cup orange juice

¾ teaspoon cinnamon

6 tablespoons sugar

1. In small bowl, combine salt, pepper, vinegar, honey, and olive oil. Rub over turkey tenderloins. Place tenderloins in zipper-lock bag and freeze.

2. To make the compote, in medium saucepan, combine remaining ingredients. Bring to a boil, reduce heat, and simmer for 5 to 8 minutes until mixture thickens slightly. Cool in ice-water bath or

refrigerator, pour into zipper-lock bag, attach to turkey tenderloins, label, and freeze.

3. To thaw and reheat: Thaw turkey and compote overnight in refrigerator. Heat 2 more tablespoons olive oil in a heavy ovenproof skillet. Brown tenderloins on all sides in hot oil. Place skillet in preheated 400° oven for 25 to 30 minutes, turning turkey once, or until internal temperature registers 170°F. Let stand 10 minutes, then slice and serve with cold compote.

Turkey Spinach Crepes

These elegant crepes are perfect for the company. To serve without freezing, place in preheated 400°F oven for 55 to 60 minutes, until filling bubbles and crepes begin to brown.

Serves 6

1 onion, chopped

1 tablespoon olive oil

1 cup frozen cut-leaf spinach

2 strips sun-dried tomatoes in oil

½ cup ricotta cheese

1 cup shredded Havarti cheese

2 cups cooked, cubed turkey

½ teaspoons dried oregano leaves

12 Basic Crepes

1 (16-ounce) jar Alfredo sauce

½ cup evaporated milk

Serves 18

3 onions, chopped

3 tablespoons olive oil

3 cups frozen cut-leaf spinach

6 strips sun-dried tomatoes in oil

1½ cups ricotta cheese

3 cups shredded Havarti cheese

6 cups cooked, cubed turkey

1½ teaspoons dried oregano leaves

36 Basic Crepes

3 (16-ounce) jars Alfredo sauce

1½ cups evaporated milk

1. In skillet, sauté onion in olive oil until crisp-tender. Add spinach; cook and stir until spinach is thawed and liquid evaporates, about 5 to 6 minutes. Remove from heat and cool completely.

2. Drain sun-dried tomatoes and mince. In large bowl, mix tomatoes with cheeses, turkey, oregano, and cooled spinach mixture.

3. Place crepes, browned-side down, on work surface. Divide turkey mixture evenly among crepes. Roll up crepes and place in 13″ × 9″ baking dish. Mix Alfredo sauce and evaporated milk and pour over casserole, and then wrap, label, and freeze.

4. To reheat: Bake casserole from frozen in preheated 400°F oven for 60 to 80 minutes, until sauce bubbles and tops of crepes brown.

Sweet and Sour Meatballs

To serve immediately, combine all sauce ingredients and bring to a boil. Reduce heat, add cooked meatballs, cover, and simmer for 7 to 9 minutes or until meatballs are hot and sauce is slightly thickened.

Serves 8–10

1 pound ground beef

1 egg

½ cup grated Parmesan cheese

¼ cup dry bread crumbs

¼ cup apple cider vinegar

1 (10-ounce) can condensed tomato soup

1 cup of sugar

1 (8-ounce) can pineapple tidbits, undrained

Serves 24–30

3 pounds ground beef

3 eggs

1½ cups grated Parmesan cheese

¾ cup dry bread crumbs

¾ cup apple cider vinegar

3 (10-ounce) cans condensed tomato soup

1 cup of sugar

3 (8-ounce) cans pineapple tidbits, undrained

1. Preheat oven to 350°F. In medium bowl, combine ground beef, egg, cheese, and bread crumbs and mix well to blend. Form into 1-inch meatballs and place on baking sheet. Bake at 350°F for 20 to 25

minutes or until no longer pink in center. Chill meatballs in refrigerator until thoroughly cold.

2. In a medium bowl, combine vinegar, soup, sugar, and pineapple tidbits and juice. Mix well and pour into a 1-gallon-size zipper-lock freezer bag. Add meatballs, seal bag, and turn gently to mix. Label bag and freeze.

3. To thaw and reheat: Thaw overnight in refrigerator. Pour meatballs and sauce into a large skillet and cook over medium heat until sauce comes to a boil. Reduce heat, cover, and simmer meatballs for 8 to 10 minutes or until thoroughly heated, stirring occasionally.

Jalapeno Pops

To serve immediately, heat oil to 375°F. Fry peppers, a few at a time, until golden brown, about 4 to 6 minutes. Drain on paper towels and serve.

Makes 24

24 small jalapeno peppers

2 cups grated Swiss cheese

1 (8-ounce) package cream cheese, softened

1 cup flour

½ teaspoon salt

1 egg, beaten

1 cup ginger ale

3 tablespoons cornstarch

Makes 72

72 small jalapeno peppers

6 cups grated Swiss cheese

3 (8-ounce) packages cream cheese, softened

3 cups flour

1½ teaspoons salt

3 eggs, beaten

2 cups ginger ale

9 tablespoons cornstarch

1. Cut slit inside of peppers and gently remove seeds and membranes. Combine Swiss cheese and cream cheese in medium bowl and blend well. Stuff peppers with cheese mixture and press gently to seal.

2. In a small bowl, combine flour, salt, egg, and ginger ale and mix until a thick batter forms. Put cornstarch in another small bowl. Dip each stuffed pepper in cornstarch and shake off excess.

Dip each pepper in batter and hold over the bowl a few seconds for excess batter to drip off.

Flash freeze peppers in a single layer on the baking sheet. When frozen solid, pack in rigid containers, with waxed paper separating layers. Label peppers and freeze.

3. To reheat: Preheat oven to 400°F. Place frozen peppers on baking sheet and bake at 400°F for 20 to 30 minutes or until brown, crisp, and thoroughly heated.

Cheesy Quesadillas

To serve immediately, simply cut the stuffed tortillas into wedges after baking. Let quesadillas cool 2 to 3 minutes and serve.

Makes 5

1 cup oil-packed sun-dried tomatoes

1 cup grated sharp Cheddar cheese

2 cups grated pepper jack cheese

½ cup grated Parmesan cheese

1 teaspoon dried oregano

1 tablespoon olive oil

10 (10-inch) flour tortillas

Makes 15

3 cups oil-packed sun-dried tomatoes

3 cups grated sharp Cheddar cheese

6 cups grated pepper jack cheese

1½ cups grated Parmesan cheese

1 tablespoon dried oregano

3 tablespoons olive oil

30 (10-inch) flour tortillas

1. Preheat oven to 400°F. Chop sun-dried tomatoes and reserve oil. In medium bowl, combine cheeses, oregano, olive oil, and chopped tomatoes and mix well. Place cheese mixture on 5 tortillas and cover with the other 5. Brush stuffed tortillas on both sides with reserved

oil and place on baking sheets. Bake at 400°F for 25 to 35 minutes or until tortillas are golden and cheese is melted.

2. Cool completely in refrigerator, then cut each stuffed tortilla into six wedges. Wrap, label, and freeze.

3. To reheat: Place frozen wedges on cookie sheet and bake at 400°F for 7 to 12 minutes, until quesadillas are hot and cheese is melted.

Spicy Snack Mix

To serve immediately, let the snack mix cool for 30 to 35 minutes after baking, and serve.

Serves 8–10

2 cups salted mixed nuts

2 cups small pretzels

2 cups potato sticks

½ cup butter, melted

3 tablespoons Worcestershire sauce

2 teaspoons dried Italian seasoning

½ teaspoon crushed red pepper flakes

1 teaspoon white pepper

Serves 24–30

6 cups salted mixed nuts

6 cups small pretzels

6 cups potato sticks

1½ cups butter, melted

9 tablespoons Worcestershire sauce

6 teaspoons dried Italian seasoning

1½ teaspoons crushed red pepper flakes

1 teaspoon white pepper

1. Preheat oven to 300ºF. Pour nuts, pretzels, and potato sticks onto two cookie sheets with sides.

In small saucepan, combine melted butter with remaining ingredients. Drizzle over the nut mixture. Toss to coat. Bake at 300ºF for 20 to 25 minutes, or until mixture is glazed and fragrant, stirring once during baking.

2. Cool snack mix and pack into zipper-lock bags. Label bags and freeze.

3. To thaw and reheat: Thaw at room temperature for 1 to 3 hours. Spread on baking sheet and reheat in 300ºF oven for 5 to 8 minutes, until crisp.

Tiny Filled Puffs

Slice off the top of these tiny puffs and fill them with a mixture of mayonnaise, chopped ham, cubed cheese, and dried basil. Any sandwich filling could be used in these easy little puffs.

Makes about 30

1 cup of water

½ cup butter

½ teaspoon salt

1 cup flour

3 eggs

½ cup grated Parmesan cheese

1 tablespoon dried chives

Makes about 90

3 cups of water

1½ cups butter

1½ teaspoons salt

3 cups flour

9 eggs

1½ cups grated Parmesan cheese

3 tablespoons dried chives

1. Preheat oven to 375°F. Line baking sheet with parchment paper and set aside. In heavy saucepan, combine water and butter. Bring to a rolling boil that cannot be stirred down. Add salt and flour all at once. Cook and stir over medium heat until dough forms a ball and cleans sides of pan.

Remove from heat and beat in eggs, one at a time, until well combined. Stir in cheese and chives.

2. Drop dough by teaspoons onto the prepared baking sheet. Bake at 375°F for 18 to 22 minutes or until dough is puffed, golden brown, and firm. Remove from baking sheet and cool on wire rack.

3. Flash freeze puffs in a single layer on the baking sheet. Then carefully pack into rigid containers. Label puffs and freeze.

4. To reheat: Place frozen puffs on the baking sheet. Bake in preheated 400°F oven for 5 to 8 minutes, until hot. Let cool slightly, then cut puffs in half and fill with desired filling.

Beefy Enchiladas

To serve immediately, sprinkle with cheese and bake casserole at 350°F for 20 to 25 minutes until thoroughly heated and bubbling around edges.

Serves 4

1 pound ground beef

1 onion, chopped

1 jalapeno pepper, seeded and minced

1 (16-ounce) can refried beans

1 (8-ounce) can tomato sauce

1 teaspoon cumin

8 flour tortillas

1 (20-ounce) can enchilada sauce

1 cup shredded Cheddar cheese

Serves 12

3 pounds ground beef

3 onions, chopped

3 jalapeno peppers, seeded and minced

3 (16-ounce) cans refried beans

3 (8-ounce) cans tomato sauce

1 tablespoon cumin

24 flour tortillas

3 (20-ounce) cans enchilada sauce

3 cups shredded Cheddar cheese

1. In heavy skillet, cook ground beef with onions and jalapenos until beef is thoroughly cooked.

Drain well. Stir in refried beans, tomato sauce, and cumin. Blend well and simmer, uncovered, for 15 minutes.

2. Stack tortillas and wrap in foil. Place in 350°F oven for 5 minutes to soften.

3. Pour ½ cup enchilada sauce in bottom of a 9″ × 9″ baking dish. Divide beef filling among tortillas and roll-up. Place stuffed tortillas in a baking dish. Cover with remaining enchilada

4. Cool enchiladas in the refrigerator, wrap, seal, label, attach zipper-lock bag containing cheese and freeze.

5. To thaw and reheat: Thaw overnight in refrigerator. Sprinkle with cheese and bake at 350°F for 30 to 35 minutes, until casserole is hot in center and bubbling around the edges.

Stuffed Manicotti

To serve immediately, sprinkle casserole with cheese and bake at 350°F for25 to 35 minutes or until bubbly and cheese is melted.

Serves 4–6

1 pound ground beef

1 onion, chopped

1 cup chopped mushrooms

1 cup bread crumbs

¼ cup milk

1 egg

½ cup grated Parmesan cheese

1 teaspoon pepper

8 manicotti shells

1 (14-ounce) jar pasta sauce

1 cup grated mozzarella cheese

½ cup grated Parmesan cheese

Serves 12–18

3 pounds ground beef

3 onions, chopped

3 cups chopped mushrooms

3 cups bread crumbs

¾ cup milk

3 eggs

1½ cups grated Parmesan cheese

1 teaspoon pepper

24 manicotti shells

3 (14-ounce) jars pasta sauce

3 cups grated mozzarella cheese

1½ cups grated Parmesan cheese

1. Brown ground beef with onion in large skillet. Drain well, then add mushrooms. Cook and stir 4 to 5 minutes longer, until mushrooms are tender. Remove from heat and add bread crumbs, milk, egg, first quantity of Parmesan cheese, and pepper. Mix well.

2. Boil manicotti shells as directed on package; drain and rinse with cold water. Place on parchment-lined cookie sheets. Stuff each shell with beef mixture.

3. Spread ½ cup pasta sauce in bottom of 9" × 9" baking dish. Top with stuffed manicotti noodles.

Cover with remaining sauce. Chill in refrigerator, then wrap, attach the bag of mixed mozzarella and

Parmesan, label, and freeze.

4. To thaw and reheat: Thaw overnight in refrigerator. Cover and bake at 350°F for 20 to 30 minutes or until hot. Uncover, sprinkle with cheeses, and bake 10 to 15 minutes longer, until casserole bubbles and cheese is melted.

Apple Meatloaf

Grated apples and applesauce make this meatloaf wonderfully moist and add great flavor. To serve immediately, bake as directed, remove from oven, let stand 10 minutes, and then slice.

Serves 4

1 pound ground beef

¼ cup applesauce

½ cup grated apple

½ cup soft bread crumbs

1 egg

½ cup apple cider

2 tablespoons mustard

1 tablespoon brown sugar

Serves 12

3 pounds ground beef

¾ cup applesauce

1½ cups grated apple

1½ cups soft bread crumbs

3 eggs

1½ cups apple cider

6 tablespoons mustard

3 tablespoons brown sugar

1. Preheat oven to 350ºF. In large bowl, combine ground beef, applesauce, grated apple, bread crumbs, and egg. Form into loaf shape and place on broiler pan. Bake at 350ºF for 30 minutes.

2. Combine apple cider, mustard, and brown sugar in small bowl. Baste meatloaf with half of this mixture and bake 20 minutes longer. Baste with remaining mixture and bake for another 15 to 20 minutes, until meatloaf registers 160ºF in center. Cool in refrigerator; wrap, pack, and freeze.

3. To thaw and reheat: Thaw overnight in refrigerator. When thawed, slice meatloaf, place in baking dish and pour ½ cup apple

juice over loaf. Bake at 375°F for 20 to 25 minutes, until meat is thoroughly heated.

To reheat from frozen: Unwrap loaf and place on broiler pan. Bake at 350°F for 1½ hours, until internal temperature registers 155°F, basting occasionally with apple juice.

Goulash

To serve this old-fashioned dish immediately, cook beef mixture and cook pasta until al dente; drain, but don't rinse. Add pasta to beef mixture. Simmer for 10 to 75 minutes, until flavors are blended.

Serves 4

1 pound ground beef

1 onion, chopped

1 (10-ounce) can condensed tomato soup

1 green bell pepper, chopped

1 (8-ounce) can tomato sauce

1 (14-ounce) can diced tomatoes, undrained

2 cups penne pasta

Serves 12

3 pounds ground beef

3 onions, chopped

3 (10-ounce) cans condensed tomato soup

3 green bell peppers, chopped

3 (8-ounce) cans tomato sauce

3 (14-ounce) cans diced tomatoes, undrained

6 cups penne pasta

1. In large skillet, cook ground beef with onion until beef is browned and onion is tender. Drain well. Add soup, green pepper, tomato sauce, and undrained tomatoes. Stir well and simmer, uncovered, for 10 minutes to blend flavors.

2. Cook pasta until almost al dente. Drain and rinse with cold water. Stir pasta into mixture in skillet. Cool mixture in refrigerator. Pack, label, and freeze.

3. To thaw and reheat: Thaw overnight in refrigerator. Pour into skillet and add ¼ cup water if necessary. Heat mixture until bubbly and serve.

Mexican Pizza

To serve immediately, spread each prebaked crust with sauce, top with cheese, and bake at 400°F for 20 to 25 minutes until cheese begins to brown.

Serves 8

2 cans refrigerated pizza dough

2 pounds ground beef

1 onion, chopped

2 cloves garlic, chopped

1 (16-ounce) can refried beans

1 (6-ounce) can tomato paste

1 cup of water

1 (12-ounce) jar salsa

1 (4-ounce) can green chilies, drained

3 cups shredded mozzarella cheese

2 cups shredded Cheddar cheese

Serves 24

6 cans refrigerated pizza dough

6 pounds ground beef

3 onions, chopped

6 cloves garlic, chopped

3 (16-ounce) cans refried beans

3 (6-ounce) cans tomato paste

1 cup of water

3 (12-ounce) jars salsa

3 (4-ounce) cans green chilies, drained

9 cups shredded mozzarella cheese

6 cups shredded Cheddar cheese

1. Roll out and prebake each pizza crust at 400°F for 10 minutes or until lightly browned. Set aside.

2. Brown ground beef with onions and garlic in heavy skillet. Drain well and add refried beans, tomato paste, water, salsa, and green chilies. Stir to combine. Simmer, uncovered, for 10 minutes to blend flavors.

3. Divide sauce among pizzas and spread evenly over each crust. Cool in refrigerator; then wrap, attach bags of mozzarella and Cheddar cheese, label, and freeze.

4. To reheat: Bake frozen pizzas at 400°F for 12 to 18 minutes until hot. Sprinkle with cheeses and bake 10 to 15 minutes longer, until cheese bubbles and begins to brown.

Beef and Potato Pie

To serve this savory old-fashioned pie immediately, bake as directed and do not refrigerate. Let stand 10 minutes before slicing.

Serves 6

9-inch Pie Crust

1 pound ground beef

1 onion, chopped

2 cloves garlic, chopped

2 cups frozen hash brown potatoes, thawed

2 tablespoons tomato paste

¼ cup ketchup

¼ cup of water

½ teaspoon oregano

2 tablespoons flour

1½ cups cottage cheese

3 eggs

2 tablespoons flour

3 tablespoons Parmesan cheese

Serves 18

3 9-inch Pie Crusts

3 pounds ground beef

3 onions, chopped

6 cloves garlic, chopped

6 cups frozen hash brown potatoes, thawed

6 tablespoons tomato paste

¾ cup ketchup

¾ cup of water

1½ teaspoons oregano

6 tablespoons flour

4½ cups cottage cheese

9 eggs

6 tablespoons flour

9 tablespoons Parmesan cheese

1. Preheat oven to 400°. Bake unfilled pie crust for 5 to 6 minutes, until set. In large skillet, sauté ground beef with onion and garlic until browned. Drain well. Add drained hash browns, tomato paste, ketchup, water, oregano, and first amount of flour; stir. Simmer for 10 to 15 minutes, until thickened. Pour into prebaked pie crust.

2. In medium bowl, combine cottage cheese, eggs, remaining flour, and Parmesan cheese and beat well with a wire whisk. Pour over meat mixture. Bake pie at 350°F for 25 to 30 minutes, until topping is puffed, set, and beginning to brown. Cool pie in refrigerator, and wrap, label, and freeze.

3. To thaw and reheat: Let pie thaw in refrigerator overnight. Bake at 350ºF for 30 to 35 minutes (cover edges of pie crust with foil if browning too fast), until thoroughly heated.

Italian Meatballs

You can use these delicious meatballs immediately by mixing with gravy and serving over noodles, or adding some pasta sauce and making a sandwich. The possibilities are endless!

Serves 4

2 tablespoons olive oil

1 onion, finely chopped

1 pound ground beef

½ cup chopped prosciutto ham

½ cup dried Italian bread crumbs

1 egg

1 teaspoon dried Italian seasoning

¼ cup milk

Serves 12

6 tablespoons olive oil

3 onions, finely chopped

3 pounds ground beef

1½ cups chopped prosciutto ham

1½ cups dried Italian bread crumbs

3 eggs

1 tablespoon dried Italian seasoning

¾ cup milk

1. In medium skillet, heat olive oil over medium heat. Sauté onion until crisp-tender.

2. In large bowl, combine cooked onion with all other ingredients and mix well to combine. Form into 24 to 30 meatballs. Place meatballs on the baking sheet. Bake at 350°F for 20 to 30 minutes, until fully cooked.

3. Place meatballs on another baking sheet and flash freeze. When meatballs are frozen, package them in a zipper-lock bag. Label bag and freeze.

4. To reheat: Bake frozen meatballs at 350°F for 10 to 12 minutes until hot, or add to Slow Cooker recipes and cook 7 to 8 hours on low.

Beef and Ziti

To serve immediately, combine ground beef sauce with ziti and pour it into a 2-quart casserole. Sprinkle with cheese and bake at 375°F for 20 to 25 minutes or until cheese melts.

Serves 4

1 pound ground beef

1 onion, chopped

2 cloves garlic, chopped

1 (14-ounce) can diced tomatoes, undrained

1 (10-ounce) can cream of potato soup

1 (8-ounce) can tomato sauce

1 teaspoon dried basil leaves

2 cups ziti pasta

2 cups shredded Colby-jack cheese

Serves 12

3 pounds ground beef

3 onions, chopped

6 cloves garlic, chopped

3 (14-ounce) cans diced tomatoes, undrained

3 (10-ounce) cans cream of potato soup

3 (8-ounce) cans tomato sauce

1 tablespoon dried basil leaves

6 cups ziti pasta

6 cups shredded Colby-jack cheese

1. Brown ground beef with onion and garlic in heavy skillet. Drain well. Add undrained tomatoes, soup, tomato sauce, and basil. Cover and simmer for 10 minutes.

2. Meanwhile, cook ziti as directed on package until almost done; drain and add to skillet. Stir well, then chill in refrigerator or ice-water bath. Pack into zipper-lock bags, attach a bag of shredded cheese, label, and freeze.

3. To thaw and reheat: Thaw overnight in refrigerator. Pour into a 2-quart casserole dish and sprinkle with cheese. Bake at 350°F for 20 to 25 minutes, until bubbly and thoroughly heated.

Cincinnati Chili

To serve immediately, break spaghetti in half and add to cooked chili; simmer for 8 to 10 minutes or until pasta is al dente Garnish with grated cheese and chopped onions.

Serves 6

1½ pounds ground beef

1 onion, chopped

3 cloves garlic, minced

1 (14-ounce) can diced tomatoes, undrained

1 (6-ounce) can tomato paste

1 (10-ounce) can condensed beef broth

3 cups of water

1 tablespoon apple cider vinegar

2 (16-ounce) cans kidney beans, drained

2 tablespoons chili powder

½ teaspoon cumin

½ teaspoon allspice

1 (6-ounce) package

spaghetti pasta

Serves 18

4½ pounds ground beef

3 onions, chopped

9 cloves garlic, minced

3 (14-ounce) cans diced tomatoes, undrained

3 (6-ounce) cans tomato paste

3 (10-ounce) cans condensed beef broth

9 cups of water

3 tablespoons apple cider vinegar

6 (16-ounce) cans kidney beans, drained

6 tablespoons chili powder

1½ teaspoons cumin

1½ teaspoons allspice

3 (6-ounce) packages spaghetti pasta

1. In large stockpot, cook ground beef, onion, and garlic until beef is browned. Drain off fat. Add remaining ingredients except spaghetti. Bring to a boil, reduce heat, and simmer for 20 to 30 minutes. Cool chili in the refrigerator or ice-water bath.

2. Pour chili into rigid containers, wrap, label, and freeze. Reserve pasta in the pantry.

3. To thaw and reheat: Thaw chili overnight in refrigerator. Place in saucepan and bring to a boil. Reduce heat and simmer for 10 to 15 minutes or until thoroughly heated. Break spaghetti in half and add to pot, making sure pasta is covered with liquid. Simmer for 8 to 12 minutes or until pasta is tender.

Chunky Spaghetti Sauce

You can serve this sauce immediately after letting it simmer for about 30 minutes to blend flavors. Cook spaghetti or linguine pasta until al dente, drain, and pour sauce over pasta.

Serves 4

1 pound ground beef

2 onions, chopped

4 cloves garlic, chopped

2 (14-ounce) cans diced tomatoes, undrained

1 (6-ounce) can tomato paste

1 (10-ounce) can condensed beef broth

1 (4-ounce) jar sliced mushrooms, undrained

1 teaspoon red pepper flakes

2 teaspoons sugar

Serves 12

3 pounds ground beef

6 onions, chopped

12 cloves garlic, chopped

6 (14-ounce) cans diced tomatoes, undrained

3 (6-ounce) cans tomato paste

3 (10-ounce) cans condensed beef broth

3 (4-ounce) jars sliced mushrooms, undrained

1teaspoon red pepper flakes

2 tablespoons sugar

1. Brown ground beef, onions, and garlic in large skillet. Drain well, then add remaining ingredients. Bring to a boil, then partially cover the pan and simmer over low heat for 25 to 30 minutes to blend flavors, stirring frequently.

2. Cool sauce in refrigerator or ice-water bath, then portion into rigid containers, wrap, label, and freeze.

3. To thaw and reheat: Thaw sauce in refrigerator overnight. Reheat in saucepan until bubbly, stirring frequently. Serve over hot cooked pasta and top with grated Parmesan cheese.

Spaghetti

To serve immediately, cook sauce over low heat for 30 to 40 minutes, stirring frequently, until thick. Serve sauce over pasta.

Serves 4

1 pound ground beef

1 onion, chopped

3 cloves garlic, minced

1 carrot, grated

1 teaspoon dried basil leaves

¼ teaspoon salt

1 (26-ounce) jar pasta sauce

1 (8-ounce) package spaghetti pasta

½ cup grated Parmesan cheese

Serves 12

3 pounds ground beef

3 onions, chopped

9 cloves garlic, minced

3 carrots, grated

1 tablespoon dried basil leaves

¾ teaspoon salt

3 (26-ounce) jars pasta sauce

3 (8-ounce) packages spaghetti pasta

1½ cups grated Parmesan cheese

1. Brown ground beef with onion and garlic in heavy skillet over medium heat. Drain well, and then add carrot, basil, salt, and pasta sauce. Simmer for 10 to 15 minutes; then cool sauce in fridge, pour into 1-gallon zipper-lock bag, attach 1-pint zipper-lock bag filled with cheese, label, and freeze. Reserve pasta in the pantry.

2. To thaw and reheat: Thaw overnight in refrigerator. Pour sauce into a heavy saucepan and add ¼ cup water. Heat, stirring frequently, until sauce comes to a boil. Cook pasta according to package directions, drain, and serve with hot sauce and grated cheese.

Meatball Veggie Casserole

To serve immediately, after returning meatballs to skillet with vegetables, simmer another 5 to 10 minutes. Assemble and bake as directed until casserole bubbles and potatoes begin to brown.

Serves 4

1 pound lean ground beef

¼ cup dry bread crumbs

3 tablespoons milk

1 egg

½ teaspoon salt

1 teaspoon pepper

2 tablespoons olive oil

1 onion, chopped

1 cup cut green beans

1 cup chopped carrots

1 cup chopped broccoli

1 (14-ounce) can diced tomatoes, undrained

2 tablespoons flour

2 cups mashed potatoes

Serves 12

3 pounds lean ground beef

¾ cup dry bread crumbs

9 tablespoons milk

3 eggs

1½ teaspoons salt

teaspoon pepper

6 tablespoons olive oil

3 onions, chopped

3 cups cut green beans

3 cups chopped carrots

3 cups chopped broccoli

3 (14-ounce) cans diced tomatoes, undrained

6 tablespoons flour

6 cups mashed potatoes

1. In large bowl, combine beef, bread crumbs, milk, egg, salt, and pepper and mix gently. Form into 24 meatballs. In large skillet, heat olive oil and sauté meatballs on all sides until brown.
Remove meatballs from pan as they cook and refrigerate.

2. In drippings remaining in skillet, sauté onions, beans, carrots, and broccoli until crisp-tender. Drain liquid from diced tomatoes and mix liquid with flour until smooth. Add tomatoes and flour mixture to pan. Simmer for 10 minutes. Add meatballs to skillet, stir, and remove from heat.

3. Chill mixture in refrigerator or ice-water bath. Place in 9″ × 9″ square baking dish and top with mashed potatoes. Wrap, label, and freeze.

4. To thaw and reheat: Thaw casserole overnight in refrigerator. Bake at 350°F for 20 to 30 minutes, until casserole is thoroughly heated and potatoes begin to brown.

Meatball Pot Pie

To serve immediately, combine soup, milk, vegetables, and cooked meatballs in skillet.

Cook over medium heat, stirring frequently, for 10 minutes. Place in pie plate, cover with pastry, and bake at 375°F for 30 to 40 minutes, until done.

Serves 6

1 pound lean ground beef

¼ cup dry bread crumbs

3 tablespoons milk

1 egg

½ teaspoon salt

½ teaspoon pepper

2 tablespoons olive oil

1 (10-ounce) can cream of celery soup

½ cup evaporated milk

2 cups frozen mixed vegetables

19-inch Pie Crust

Serves 18

3 pounds lean ground beef

¾ cup dry bread crumbs

9 tablespoons milk

3 eggs

1½ teaspoons salt

1 teaspoon pepper

6 tablespoons olive oil

3 (10-ounce) cans cream of celery soup

1½ cups evaporated milk

6 cups of frozen mixed vegetables

3 9-inch Pie Crusts

1. In large bowl, combine ground beef, bread crumbs, milk, egg, salt, and pepper and mix gently. Form into 24 meatballs. Heat olive oil in heavy skillet and brown meatballs, turning occasionally, until browned and fully cooked. Drain on paper towels. Cool meatballs in the refrigerator.

2. In 9-inch deep-dish pie plate, combine soup, milk, and vegetables. Add cold meatballs and mix gently. Place pastry on top of mixture, seal edges, and flute. Cut slits in a decorative pattern in the top crust. Wrap, label, and freeze.

3. To thaw and reheat: Thaw pie overnight in refrigerator. Bake at 375°F for 35 to 45 minutes, until pie is thoroughly heated and bubbling and crust is brown.

Creamy Swiss Meatballs

To serve immediately, pour meatball and sauce mixture into 9" square baking dish. Bake at 375°F for 20 to 30 minutes, until bubbly and thoroughly heated.

Serves 4

1 pound lean ground beef

¼ cup dry bread crumbs

3 tablespoons milk

1 egg

½ teaspoon celery salt

1 teaspoon pepper

½ cup grated Swiss cheese

2 tablespoons olive oil

1 cup of brown rice

1 leek, chopped

2 cloves garlic, chopped

1 (10-ounce) jar Alfredo sauce

½ cup evaporated milk

½ cup grated Parmesan cheese

1 cup grated Swiss cheese

Serves 12

3 pounds lean ground beef

¾ cup dry bread crumbs

9 tablespoons milk

3 eggs

1½ teaspoons celery salt

1 teaspoon pepper

1½ cups grated Swiss cheese

6 tablespoons olive oil

3 cups brown rice

3 leeks, chopped

6 cloves garlic, chopped

3 (10-ounce) jars Alfredo sauce

1½ cups evaporated milk

1½ cups grated Parmesan cheese

3 cups grated Swiss cheese

1. In large bowl, combine beef, bread crumbs, milk, egg, celery salt, pepper, and first quantity of

Swiss cheese and mix gently. Form into 20 meatballs. Heat olive oil in large skillet and brown meatballs on all sides, turning occasionally.

2. Meanwhile, cook rice as directed on package, undercooking slightly. When meatballs are done, remove from skillet. Sauté leek and garlic in pan drippings until crisp-tender. Add Alfredo sauce, milk, remaining cheeses, browned meatballs, and cooked rice and mix gently.

3. Pour mixture into 9″ × 9″ baking dish; wrap, label, and freeze.

4. To thaw and reheat: Thaw casserole overnight in refrigerator. Bake at 375°F for 25 to 35 minutes, until casserole bubbles and meatballs are hot in center.

Mom's Favorite Meatloaf

The mushrooms and oatmeal in this meatloaf recipe add moistness and flavor. To serve immediately, bake meatloaf as directed. Cover with foil and let stand 10 minutes before slicing.

Serves 4–6

2 pounds ground beef

½ pound ground pork

1 onion, minced

½ cup minced mushrooms

1 egg

½ cup quick oatmeal

½ cup tomato sauce

1 teaspoon seasoned salt

1 teaspoon pepper

½ cup Beef Broth

½ cup tomato sauce

1 tablespoon mustard

Serves 12–18

6 pounds ground beef

1½ pounds ground pork

3 onions, minced

1½ cups minced mushrooms

3 eggs

1½ cups quick oatmeal

1½ cups tomato sauce

1 tablespoon seasoned salt

teaspoon pepper

1½ cups Beef Broth

1½ cups tomato sauce

3 tablespoons mustard

1. In large bowl, combine all ingredients except final tomato sauce and mustard and mix gently but thoroughly. Form into large

meatloaf and place on broiling rack. Combine remaining tomato sauce and mustard in small bowl and pour over meatloaf. Bake at 350°F for 55 to 65 minutes, until internal temperature registers 160°F, basting occasionally with pan drippings.

2. Cool meatloaf completely in refrigerator, then wrap, label, and freeze.

3. To thaw: Thaw overnight in refrigerator. Since meatloaf is fully cooked, it can be served cold.

To reheat: Slice meatloaf, place in baking dish, and pour ½ cup of beef broth or beef gravy over loaf. Cover dish and bake at 375°F for 20 to 25 minutes until meat is thoroughly heated.

To reheat from frozen: Unwrap loaf and place on broiler pan. Bake at 350°F for 1½ hours, until internal temperature registers 155°F, basting occasionally with ½ cup beef broth.

Beefy Bean Burritos

These easy and delicious burritos can be made hot or mild, depending on the salsa and peppers. To serve immediately, spread hot filling on warmed flour tortillas, sprinkle with cheese, and roll-up.

Serves 4

1 pound ground beef

1 onion, chopped

4 cloves garlic, minced

1 (16-ounce) can refried beans

1 (14-ounce) jar chunky salsa

1 tablespoon chili powder

1 teaspoon cumin

1 (4-ounce) can chopped jalapeno peppers

2 cups shredded Cheddar cheese

12 flour tortillas

Serves 12

3 pounds ground beef

3 onions, chopped

12 cloves garlic, minced

3 (16 ounce) cans refried beans

3 (14 ounce) jars chunky salsa

3 tablespoons chili powder

1 tablespoon cumin

3 (4 ounce) cans chopped jalapeno peppers

6 cups shredded Cheddar cheese

36 flour tortillas

1. In large skillet, brown ground beef with onions and garlic until beef is browned. Drain well.

Add remaining ingredients except for cheese and tortillas. Stir to combine. Simmer for 10 to 15 minutes to blend flavors.

2. Cool mixture in refrigerator or ice-water bath. Pack into zipper-lock bags, label, attach a bag with cheese and bag with tortillas and freeze. To assemble burritos before freezing, spread chilled filling

on tortillas and top with cheese; roll to enclose filling. Flash freeze on a baking sheet, then wrap individually, package, and place in freezer.

3. To thaw and reheat unassembled burritos: Thaw overnight in refrigerator. Place meat mixture in skillet and cook over medium heat, stirring frequently, until hot. Wrap tortillas in foil and place in 350°F oven for 10 to 12 minutes, until hot. Assemble burritos and serve.

To reheat assembled burritos: Wrap each frozen burrito in a microwave-safe paper towel.

Microwave, one at a time, on medium for 2 minutes, then rotate and microwave on high for 1 to 2 minutes longer, until hot. Or unwrap and bake frozen burritos at 400°F for 15 to 25 minutes, until hot and crisp.

Wild Rice Meatloaf

To serve immediately, bake at 350°F for 60 to 75 minutes, until internal temperature registers 160°F. Let meatloaf stand, covered, 10 minutes before serving.

Serves 6

½ cup wild rice

1 onion, finely chopped

1 clove garlic, minced

1 tablespoon olive oil

¼ cup dried bread crumbs

2 eggs, beaten

½ cup milk

1 tablespoon mustard

1 teaspoon salt

¼ teaspoon pepper

¼ cup grated Parmesan cheese

1 teaspoon dried thyme leaves

1 teaspoon dried basil leaves

1 pound lean ground beef

1 pound lean ground pork

½ cup Beef Broth or gravy

Serves 18

1½ cups wild rice

3 onions, finely chopped

3 cloves garlic, minced

3 tablespoons olive oil

¾ cup dried bread crumbs

6 eggs, beaten

1½ cups milk

3 tablespoons mustard

2 teaspoons salt

¾ teaspoon pepper

¾ cup grated Parmesan cheese

1 tablespoon dried thyme leaves

1 tablespoon dried basil leaves

3 pounds lean ground beef

3 pounds lean ground pork

1½ cups Beef Broth or gravy

1. Cook wild rice according to package directions until tender but still firm; drain. In large skillet, sauté onion and garlic in olive oil until almost crisp-tender.

2. In large bowl, combine cooked wild rice, sautéed onion and garlic, bread crumbs, eggs, milk, mustard, salt, pepper, Parmesan cheese, thyme, and basil; mix well. Add meat and mix gently but thoroughly with hands.

3. Form into oblong shape on broiler pan. Cover and bake at 350°F for 60 minutes. Remove cover and bake for 15 to 25 minutes longer until internal temperature registers 165°F. Cool in refrigerator; then wrap, label, and freeze. Reserve beef broth or gravy in the freezer.

4. To thaw: Thaw overnight in refrigerator. Since meatloaf is fully cooked, it can be served cold.

To reheat: Slice meatloaf, place in baking dish, and pour ½ cup of beef broth or beef gravy over loaf. Cover dish and bake at 375½F for 20 to 25 minutes, until meat is thoroughly heated.

To reheat from frozen: Unwrap loaf and place on broiler pan. Bake at 350°F for 1½ hours until internal temperature registers 155°F, basting occasionally with ° cup beef broth.

Easy Lasagna

To serve without freezing, cover tightly with foil and bake at 350½F for 1 hour.

Uncover, sprinkle with cheese, and bake another 10 to 75 minutes, until casserole is bubbling and cheese browns.

Serves 6

1 pound ground beef

1 onion, chopped

3 cloves garlic, minced

1 (26-ounce) jar pasta sauce

1 cup of water

2 cups ricotta cheese

1 (3-ounce) package cream cheese

1 egg

1 teaspoon salt

¼ teaspoon pepper

2 cups shredded mozzarella cheese

9 uncooked lasagna noodles

1 cup grated Parmesan cheese

Serves 18

3 pounds ground beef

3 onions, chopped

9 cloves garlic, minced

3 (26-ounce) jars pasta sauce

3 cups of water

6 cups ricotta cheese

3 (3-ounce) packages cream cheese

3 eggs

2 teaspoons salt

¾ teaspoon pepper

6 cups shredded mozzarella cheese

27 uncooked lasagna noodles

3 cups grated Parmesan cheese

1. In large skillet, brown ground beef with onion and garlic; drain. Add pasta sauce and water; mix well.

2. In large bowl, combine ricotta, cream cheese, egg, salt, and pepper and mix well. Stir in mozzarella cheese.

3. In 13" × 9" baking dish lined with freezer wrap, place 1 cup ground beef mixture. Lay 3 uncooked lasagna noodles on top. Spread one-third of ricotta filling over noodles and top with one-third of the remaining ground beef mixture. Repeat layers twice, ending with ground beef mixture. Chill in refrigerator, then wrap and freeze until firm. Pop lasagna out of the pan, wrap again, attach a bag with 1 cup grated Parmesan cheese, label, and freeze.

4. To thaw and reheat: Unwrap lasagna and place in 13" × 9" pan; thaw overnight in refrigerator.

Bake casserole, covered, at 350°F for 60 to 75 minutes, until hot in center. Uncover, sprinkle with reserved Parmesan cheese, and bake 10 to 15 minutes longer, until pasta is tender and casserole is bubbly. Let stand 15 minutes before serving.

Cabbage Rolls

To serve immediately, bake at 375°F for 30 to 40 minutes, until sauce bubbles and rolls are thoroughly heated. Any leftover shredded cabbage can be made into coleslaw.

Serves 4

1 head green cabbage

1 pound ground beef

1 onion, chopped

3 cloves garlic, minced

1 cup cooked long-grain rice

1 tablespoon mustard

2 tablespoons ketchup

1 egg, beaten

¼ teaspoon pepper

1 (15-ounce) can tomato sauce

1 (10-ounce) can condensed tomato soup

Serves 12

3 heads green cabbage

3 pounds ground beef

3 onions, chopped

9 cloves garlic, minced

3 cups cooked long-grain rice

3 tablespoons mustard

6 tablespoons ketchup

3 eggs, beaten

¾ teaspoon pepper

3 (15-ounce) cans tomato sauce

3 (10-ounce) cans condensed tomato soup

1. Core cabbage and carefully remove 8 whole cabbage leaves from head. Soak leaves in hot water while preparing filling. Shred remaining cabbage; set aside 3 cups to use in filling.

2. Cook ground beef, onion, and garlic in heavy skillet until beef is browned and onion and garlic are tender; drain well. Remove from heat and add rice, mustard, and ketchup and mix well. Stir in egg, pepper, and shredded cabbage. Fill each cabbage leaf with filling and roll-up.

3. Line a 13″ × 9″ baking pan with freezer wrap. Pour 1 cup tomato sauce into a lined pan. Arrange cabbage rolls, seam-side down, in pan. Place any remaining filling around filled rolls. Mix together remaining tomato sauce and condensed tomato soup and pour over filled rolls. Cool in the fridge until cold; then freeze until solid. When frozen solid, pop out of pan, wrap, label, and freeze.

4. To thaw and reheat: Unwrap casserole and place in 13″ × 9″ baking pan; thaw overnight in refrigerator. Cover casserole and bake at 375ºF for 50 to 60 minutes or until hot. Remove cover and bake an additional 10 to 15 minutes, until bubbly.

Beef Stew

To serve this stew immediately, prepare as directed, but don't cool it. Add frozen potato wedges and green beans to stew and simmer for 20 to 30 minutes longer, until vegetables are tender.

Serves 4

1 pound beef round steak

2 tablespoons flour

½ teaspoon salt

teaspoon pepper

1 tablespoon olive oil

1 onion, chopped

3 cloves garlic, chopped

1 (9-ounce) bag baby carrots

1 (14-ounce) can diced tomatoes, undrained

1 (10-ounce) can condensed beef broth

1 (8-ounce) can apple juice

2 cups of water

1 (16-ounce) bag frozen potato wedges

1 cup frozen green beans

Serves 12

3 pounds beef round steak

6 tablespoons flour

1½ teaspoons salt

1 teaspoon pepper

3 tablespoons olive oil

3 onions, chopped

9 cloves garlic, chopped

3 (9-ounce) bags baby carrots

3 (14-ounce) cans diced tomatoes, undrained

3 (10-ounce) cans condensed beef broth

3 (8-ounce) cans apple juice

6 cups of water

3 (16-ounce) bags frozen potato wedges

3 cups frozen green beans

1. Cut steak into 1-inch pieces and toss with flour, salt, and pepper. In large skillet over medium-high heat, cook beef in olive oil until brown, about 2 to 3 minutes, stirring frequently. Add onion and garlic; cook and stir for 4 to 5 minutes until crisp-tender. Add baby carrots, undrained tomatoes, beef broth, apple juice, and water; stir. Bring to a boil, then cover pan and simmer for

1 to 2 hours, until beef is thoroughly cooked.

2. Cool stew in an ice-water bath or in refrigerator, pour into 1-gallon zipper-lock bag, and seal bag.

Attach bag containing frozen potatoes and frozen green beans. Label and freeze.

3. To thaw and reheat: Thaw stew in the refrigerator overnight. Keep potatoes and green beans frozen. Pour stew mixture into large saucepan and bring to a boil. Add potatoes and green beans and bring back to a boil; then reduce heat, cover, and simmer for 20 to

30 minutes, until vegetables are tender and stew is thoroughly heated.

Beef Carbonado

Beer adds great depth of flavor to this rich beef stew. To serve without freezing, keep simmering stew while you cook the frozen noodles. Drain noodles and serve with the stew.

Serves 8

2 pounds beef chuck steak

3 tablespoons flour

½ teaspoon salt

½ teaspoon pepper

2 tablespoons olive oil

2 onions, chopped

4 cloves garlic, chopped

1 (8-ounce) package mushrooms, chopped

1 (12-ounce) can beer

1 teaspoon dried thyme

3 carrots, sliced

3 cups Beef Broth

1 (16-ounce) package frozen spaetzle noodles

Serves 24

6 pounds beef chuck steak

9 tablespoons flour

1½ teaspoons salt

1 teaspoon pepper

6 tablespoons olive oil

6 onions, chopped

12 cloves garlic, chopped

3 (8-ounce) packages mushrooms, chopped

3 (12-ounce) cans beer

1 tablespoon dried thyme

9 carrots, sliced

9 cups Beef Broth

3 (16-ounce) packages frozen spaetzle noodles

1. Cut steak into 2-inch pieces. Toss with flour, salt, and pepper. Heat olive oil in large saucepan and cook steak, in batches, until browned, about 5 to 6 minutes per batch. When all the beef is browned, remove from pan and set aside. Cook onions, garlic, and mushrooms in the drippings remaining in saucepan. Cook and stir until onions are crisp-tender.

2. Return beef to saucepan along with beer, thyme, carrots, and broth. Bring to a boil; reduce heat, cover pot, and let simmer for 2 to 3 hours, until beef is cooked and vegetables are tender. Cool in an ice-water bath or in refrigerator. Pour into 2-gallon-size zipper-lock bags; attach frozen noodles, label, and freeze.

3. To thaw and reheat: Thaw stew overnight in refrigerator. Keep noodles frozen. Place stew in saucepan and add ½ cup water if necessary. Cook over medium-low heat, stirring frequently, until

thoroughly heated. Cook noodles according to package directions and serve with stew.

Beef Stroganoff

To serve immediately, mix sour cream with flour and liquid and add to stroganoff.

Simmer until thickened and serve with hot egg noodles.

Serves 4

1 pound beef sirloin steak

½ teaspoon salt

teaspoon pepper

1 tablespoon olive oil

1 tablespoon butter

1 onion, chopped

3 cloves garlic, chopped

1 (8-ounce) package mushrooms, chopped

1 (10-ounce) can condensed beef broth

1 cup of water

1 tablespoon Worcestershire sauce

1 teaspoon dried marjoram

1 cup sour cream

2 tablespoons flour

3 cups uncooked egg noodles

Serves 12

3 pounds beef sirloin steak

1½ teaspoons salt

1 teaspoon pepper

3 tablespoons olive oil

3 tablespoons butter

3 onions, chopped

9 cloves garlic, chopped

3 (8-ounce) packages mushrooms, chopped

3 (10-ounce) cans condensed beef broth

3 cups of water

3 tablespoons Worcestershire sauce

1 tablespoon dried marjoram

3 cups sour cream

6 tablespoons flour

9 cups uncooked egg noodles

1. Cut steak into 1-inch cubes and sprinkle with salt and pepper. Heat olive oil and butter in large saucepan and brown beef cubes in batches, about 4 to 5 minutes per batch. Add onions, garlic, and mushrooms to drippings in saucepan and cook until crisp-tender, stirring frequently.

2. Return beef to saucepan and add broth, water, Worcestershire sauce, and marjoram; stir. Bring
to a boil, then reduce heat, cover saucepan, and simmer for 1½ hours until beef is tender. Cool in an ice-water bath or in refrigerator.

3. Pour into 1-gallon-size zipper-lock bag; label and freeze. Reserve sour cream in the fridge, and

flour and egg noodles in the pantry.

4. To thaw and reheat: Thaw overnight in refrigerator. Pour stroganoff into saucepan and bring to a boil. In medium bowl, combine sour cream, flour, and a cup of the stroganoff liquid and beat

well with wire whisk. Stir into stroganoff and cook until thickened. Cook egg noodles as directed on package and serve with stroganoff.

Pot Roast

To serve this classic savory pot roast immediately, when beef is tender, remove from oven and let stand, covered, for 10 minutes. Slice beef and serve with vegetables and sauce.

Serves 10-12

1 (5-pound) chuck roast

1 teaspoon salt

¼ teaspoon pepper

2 teaspoons paprika

¼ cup olive oil

2 onions, chopped

4 carrots, chopped

4 cloves garlic, chopped

1½ cups Beef Broth

1 teaspoon dried marjoram leaves

1 (6-ounce) can tomato paste

Serves 30–36

3 (5-pound) chuck roasts

1 tablespoon salt

¾ teaspoon pepper

6 teaspoons paprika

¾ cup olive oil

6 onions, chopped

12 carrots, chopped

12 cloves garlic, chopped

4½ cups Beef Broth

1 tablespoon dried marjoram leaves

3 (6-ounce) cans tomato paste

1. Sprinkle roast on all sides with salt, pepper, and paprika. Heat olive oil in large skillet and brown roast on all sides, about 10 minutes total. Remove roast from skillet and place in large ovenproof casserole or Dutch oven.

2. Add onions, carrots, and garlic to drippings in skillet and cook and stir until crisp-tender. Pour beef broth, marjoram, and tomato paste into skillet. Cook and stir to loosen pan drippings for 4 to 5 minutes. Pour vegetables and sauce over roast in casserole. Cover and bake at 325°F for 3 to 4 hours, until meat is very tender.

3. Cool beef, vegetables, and sauce in an ice-water bath or refrigerator. When cold, slice beef. Place beef slices, vegetables, and sauce in 2-gallon-size zipper-lock bags. Seal bags, label, and freeze.

4. To thaw and reheat: Thaw overnight in refrigerator. Place contents of bags in heavy skillet.

Cook over medium heat, stirring occasionally, until sauce bubbles and meat and vegetables are thoroughly heated, about 10 to 15 minutes.

Mini Beef Pizzas

To serve these pizzas immediately, bake at 375°F for 75 to 20 minutes until pizza is hot, English muffin is toasted and crisp, and cheese is melted and bubbly.

Serves 4–6

1 pound round steak

2 tablespoons Worcestershire sauce

1 teaspoon pepper

1 tablespoon olive oil

12 thin slices Colby cheese

6 English muffins, split

2 cups pizza sauce

1 cup frozen peppers and onions

2 cups shredded mozzarella cheese

Serves 12–18

3 pounds round steak

6 tablespoons Worcestershire sauce

1 teaspoon pepper

3 tablespoons olive oil

36 thin slices Colby cheese

18 English muffins, split

6 cups pizza sauce

3 cups frozen peppers and onions

6 cups shredded mozzarella cheese

1. Sprinkle steak with Worcestershire sauce, pepper, and olive oil on both sides and let marinate in refrigerator for 1 to 2 hours. Remove from refrigerator and place on broiler pan. Broil 4 to 6 inches from heat for 4 to 5 minutes on each side until beef is slightly pink in center. Let steak stand at room temperature for 10 minutes. Cut steak into ½-inch cubes.

2. Place Colby cheese slices on cut sides of English muffins. Top each with 1 tablespoon of pizza sauce, then divide steak cubes among pizzas. Top with remaining pizza sauce, then peppers and onions. Sprinkle with mozzarella cheese. Wrap pizzas individually, label, and freeze.

3. To reheat: Place frozen mini-pizzas on baking sheet and bake in preheated 375°F oven for 20 to 25 minutes, until hot and bubbly.

Italian Beef and Beans

To serve this simple dinner immediately, let steaks marinate in the refrigerator for 7 to 2 hours. Then cook steaks over grill or under broiler, heating sauce in saucepan at the same time.

Serves 4

1 onion, chopped

3 cloves garlic, chopped

1 tablespoon olive oil

1 (16-ounce) can cannellini beans, drained

1 (14-ounce) can diced tomatoes, undrained

1 teaspoon dried Italian seasoning

4 sirloin steaks

3 tablespoons red wine vinegar

Serves 12

3 onions, chopped

9 cloves garlic, chopped

3 tablespoons olive oil

3 (16-ounce) cans cannellini beans, drained

3 (14-ounce) cans diced tomatoes, undrained

1 tablespoon dried Italian seasoning

12 sirloin steaks

9 tablespoons red wine vinegar

1. In heavy skillet, cook onion and garlic in olive oil over medium heat until crisp-tender. Remove from heat and add beans, undrained tomatoes, and seasoning. Pour into a zipper-lock bag. Rub steaks

with red wine vinegar and place in separate zipper-lock bag. Place both bags in a larger zipper-lock bag; then label, seal and freeze.

2. To thaw and reheat: Thaw overnight in refrigerator. Broil or grill steaks 4 to 6 inches from heat source for 4 to 5 minutes per side until medium doneness. While steak is cooking, place sauce in a heavy saucepan and cook over medium heat, stirring frequently, until sauce boils; boil for 3 to 4 minutes. Serve sauce over steak.

Sauerbraten

To serve immediately, add crushed gingersnap cookies to gravy and simmer 10 to 75 minutes until thickened. Serve over hot cooked egg noodles.

Serves 6

2-pound chuck roast

3 tablespoons olive oil

1 teaspoon salt

¼ teaspoon pepper

2 onions, chopped

½ cup red wine vinegar

½ cup red wine

1 cup Beef Broth

½ teaspoon ground cloves

1 teaspoon allspice

¼ cup brown sugar

2 stalks celery, minced

12 gingersnap cookies

3 cups egg noodles

Serves 18

6-pound chuck roast

9 tablespoons olive oil

1 tablespoon salt

¾ teaspoon pepper

6 onions, chopped

1½ cups red wine vinegar

1½ cups red wine

3 cups Beef Broth

1½ teaspoons ground cloves

¼ teaspoon allspice

¾ cup brown sugar

6 stalks celery, minced

36 gingersnap cookies

9 cups egg noodles

1. Trim excess fat off roast and cut into 1½-inch cubes. Heat olive oil in Dutch oven or large ovenproof casserole. Sprinkle meat with salt and pepper and brown on all sides over medium heat.

2. Add onions; cook and stir for 3 to 4 minutes longer to partially cook onions. Add all remaining ingredients except gingersnaps and egg noodles. Cover casserole and bring sauce to a boil. Then reduce heat to low and simmer for 2½ to 3 hours until beef is very tender.

3. Cool casserole in an ice-water bath or refrigerator. Slice beef into Mi-inch-thick slices. Place beef and sauce in gallon-size zipper-lock bags. Attach a small bag with gingersnap cookies. Label bags and freeze. Reserve egg noodles in the pantry.

4. To thaw and reheat: Thaw overnight in refrigerator. Pour meat mixture into large saucepan and bring to a simmer over medium heat. Crush gingersnap cookies and add to sauce. Cook, stirring occasionally for 10 to 12 minutes, until meat is hot and sauce has thickened. Cook noodles according to package directions and serve with sauerbraten.

Beef Barley Stew

To serve immediately, simmer stew with barley added for 30 minutes. Then add frozen green beans, bring back to a simmer, and cook 10 to 75 minutes until barley is tender.

Serves 4–6

1 pound chuck roast

3 tablespoons flour

1 teaspoon salt

¼ teaspoon pepper

1 teaspoon dried marjoram leaves

2 tablespoons olive oil

1 onion, chopped

1 leek, chopped

4 carrots, peeled and chopped

1 (8-ounce) can tomato sauce

2 cups Beef Broth

½ cup medium pearl barley

2 cups frozen green beans

Serves 12–18

3 pounds chuck roast

9 tablespoons flour

1 tablespoon salt

¾ teaspoon pepper

1 tablespoon dried marjoram leaves

6 tablespoons olive oil

3 onions, chopped

3 leeks, chopped

12 carrots, peeled and chopped

3 (8-ounce) cans tomato sauce

6 cups Beef Broth

1½ cups medium pearl barley

6 cups frozen green beans

1. Trim beef and cut into 1-inch pieces. Combine flour, salt, pepper, and marjoram on shallow plate and toss with beef to coat. Heat olive oil in large stockpot and brown beef on all sides, 5 to 6 minutes total. Then add onion, leek, and carrots. Cook and stir 4 to 5 minutes until crisp-tender.

Add tomato sauce and broth. Bring to a boil, then cover, reduce heat, and simmer for 2 hours.

2. Add barley, stir, and simmer for 30 minutes. Cool stew in ice-water bath or refrigerator, then pack into rigid containers. Attach bag with frozen green beans; then label and freeze.

3. To thaw and reheat: Thaw stew overnight in refrigerator. Keep green beans frozen. Place stew in large saucepan and bring to a simmer. After five minutes, add beans, stir, and bring back to a simmer. Simmer, stirring occasionally, for 10 to 15 minutes until stew is thoroughly heated and barley and green beans are tender.

Swiss Steak

To serve without freezing, just serve the steak when it's tender and the sauce is slightly thickened. The sauce is really perfect served over hot mashed potatoes.

Serves 6

¼ cup flour

1 teaspoon salt

teaspoon pepper

1 teaspoon paprika

2 pounds round steak

3 tablespoons olive oil

2 tablespoons butter

1 onion, sliced

2 (14-ounce) cans diced tomatoes, undrained

1 (8-ounce) can tomato sauce

½ cup Beef Broth

Serves 18

¾ cup flour

1 tablespoon salt

1 teaspoon pepper

1 tablespoon paprika

6 pounds round steak

9 tablespoons olive oil

6 tablespoons butter

3 onions, sliced

6 (14-ounce) cans diced tomatoes, undrained

3 (8-ounce) cans tomato sauce

1½ cups Beef Broth

1. Combine flour and seasonings in small bowl. Cut steak into 6 pieces. Place meat between two layers of waxed paper and pound with mallet or rolling pin to flatten. Remove the top sheet of waxed paper and sprinkle meat with half of the flour mixture. Replace waxed paper and pound flour mixture into the meat. Turn meat over and repeat on the other side with remaining flour mixture.

2. Heat olive oil and butter in large skillet and add onion. Cook and stir until crisp-tender. Then add floured steaks and cook on one side until golden, about 4 to 5 minutes. Turn steaks over and cook for 2 to 3 minutes. Add tomatoes, tomato sauce, and beef broth to skillet

and bring to a boil. Reduce heat, cover pan, and simmer for 1 to 1½ hours until steak is tender.

3. Cool steak and sauce in an ice-water bath or refrigerator. Pour into zipper-lock bags, seal, label, and freeze.

4. To thaw and reheat: Thaw overnight in refrigerator. Place steak and sauce in large skillet and cook over medium heat until steak is hot and sauce bubbles.

Stuffed Peppers

To serve immediately, don't chill tilling. Fill peppers with hot meat mixture and place in baking dish. Sprinkle with cheese and pour sauce over. Bake at 350°F for 20 to 25 minutes.

Serves 4

4 green bell peppers

½ cup medium barley

1 onion, chopped

3 cloves garlic, chopped

2 tablespoons olive oil

2 cups cooked, cubed beef

1 teaspoon salt

¼ teaspoon red pepper flakes

1 (8-ounce) can tomato sauce

1 cup shredded Cruyère cheese

1 (8-ounce) can tomato sauce

Serves 12

12 green bell peppers

1½ cups medium barley

3 onions, chopped

9 cloves garlic, chopped 6 tablespoons olive oil

6 cups cooked, cubed beef

1 tablespoon salt

¾ teaspoon red pepper flakes

3 (8-ounce) cans tomato sauce

3 cups shredded Cruyère cheese

3 (8-ounce) cans tomato sauce

1. Cut the tops off the green peppers and remove veins and seeds. Rinse well, then submerge peppers in boiling water for 2 to 3 minutes. Remove and drain upside down on kitchen towels. Chop pepper tops, discarding stem.

2. Cook barley according to package directions until almost tender. Drain well and set aside.

3. In large skillet, sauté onion and garlic in olive oil until crisp-tender; drain well. Add beef, salt, red pepper, and first can of tomato sauce; simmer for 10 minutes to blend flavors. Cool beef mixture in refrigerator or ice-water bath.

4. Stuff peppers with cooled beef mixture and sprinkle each with shredded cheese. Wrap each pepper, label, and freeze. Reserve the remaining tomato sauce in the pantry.

5. To thaw and reheat: Thaw overnight in refrigerator. Place thawed peppers in 9″ × 9″ square baking dish and pour tomato sauce over all. Bake at 350ºF for 25 to 30 minutes, until thoroughly heated, basting peppers occasionally with sauce.

Shredded Beef Tacos

To serve immediately, place shredded beef, tomatoes, and chilies in large skillet. Cook over medium heat until the mixture thickens. Heat taco shells in oven; then spoon beef mixture into shells.

Serves 4

1 pound beef chuck roast

1 teaspoon salt

1 teaspoon pepper

5 cloves garlic, slivered

3 cups of water

1 (14-ounce) can diced tomatoes, undrained

1 (4-ounce) can chopped green chilies

8 taco shells

Serves 12

3 pounds beef chuck roast

1 tablespoon salt

1 teaspoon pepper

15 cloves garlic, slivered

9 cups of water

3 (14-ounce) cans diced tomatoes, undrained

3 (4-ounce) cans chopped green chilies

24 taco shells

1. Sprinkle beef with salt and pepper. Cut small slits in beef and insert garlic slivers. Place in a large stockpot. Pour water over; then cover the stockpot and bring to a boil. Reduce heat and simmer for 1½ hours, until beef is very tender.

2. Drain beef; then cool in refrigerator. Shred the meat using two forks. Combine with tomatoes and green chilies in a zipper-lock bag. Seal bag, attach bagged taco shells, then label and freeze.

3. To thaw and reheat: Thaw overnight in refrigerator. Heat beef mixture in heavy skillet until hot, stirring occasionally, about 10 to 15 minutes. Bake taco shells in preheated 400°F oven for 4 to 5 minutes until crisp. Serve beef mixture in taco shells; garnish with lettuce, cheese, taco sauce, and sour cream.

Thai Beef Skewers

To serve skewers without freezing, marinate beef in refrigerator for 2 to 8 hours. Grill or broil 4 to 6 inches from heat, 2 to 3 minutes on each side.

Serves 3–4

1 pound beef flank steak

2 shallots, minced

4 cloves garlic, minced

1 teaspoon salt

1 teaspoon red pepper flakes

1 tablespoon grated gingerroot

¼ cup teriyaki sauce

3 tablespoons honey

2 tablespoons rice wine vinegar

Serves 12–16

3 pounds beef flank steak

6 shallots, minced

12 cloves garlic, minced

1 tablespoon salt

¾ teaspoon red pepper flakes

3 tablespoons grated ginger root

¾ cup teriyaki sauce

9 tablespoons honey

6 tablespoons rice wine vinegar

1. Partially freeze meat for 1 hour, then slice thinly across the grain into 1-inch strips. To make marinade, combine remaining ingredients in medium bowl and mix well. Add steak strips to marinade and toss to coat.

2. Thread beef onto 20 metal skewers, then place in quart-size zipper-lock bags and pour remaining marinade into bag. Seal, label, and freeze.

3. To thaw and reheat: Thaw beef overnight in refrigerator. Grill or broil 4 to 6 inches from heat source for 2 minutes on each side until beef is medium-done. Discard remaining marinade.

Don't Forget to Thaw!

Designate a special space in your refrigerator just for thawing foods. When you remove that night's dish from the refrigerator, that empty space will remind you to take another dish from the freezer and put it in the fridge for overnight thawing.

Beef Rouladen

This twist on the German classic combines bacon and brown rice in creamy beef gravy. You can serve this dish immediately with some mashed potatoes to soak up the sauce.

Serves 4–6

8 ¼-inch-thick slices bottom round steak

3 tablespoons brown mustard

½ cup of brown rice

1½ cups water

4 slices bacon

1 tablespoon butter

1 onion, chopped

3 cloves garlic, chopped

3 tablespoons flour

2 cups Beef Broth

2 tablespoons olive oil

Serves 12–18

24 ¼-inch-thick slices bottom round steak

9 tablespoons brown mustard

1½ cups brown rice

4½ cups water

12 slices bacon

3 tablespoons butter

3 onions, chopped

9 cloves garlic, chopped

9 tablespoons flour

6 cups Beef Broth

6 tablespoons olive oil

1. Spread mustard on steak slices and set aside. Cook brown rice in water for 30 to 40 minutes until almost tender. Drain if necessary and set aside. Cook bacon in large skillet over medium heat until crisp. Remove from skillet and drain on paper towels; crumble and set aside.

2. Add butter to drippings in skillet and add onions and garlic. Cook and stir over medium heat until crisp-tender. Sprinkle flour over onions and cook and stir for 2 to 3 minutes, stirring constantly. Add half of beef broth and cook until mixture thickens, about 4 to 5 minutes. Add brown rice and crumbled bacon to this mixture.

3. Divide rice mixture among the round steak slices. Roll up, enclosing filling. Use toothpicks to hold rolls closed, if necessary.

Heat olive oil in skillet and brown beef rolls on all sides over medium heat. Add remaining beef broth to skillet and bring to a boil. Cover skillet, reduce heat, and simmer beef rolls for 30 to 45 minutes, until very tender. Cool beef rolls and sauce in an ice water bath or refrigerator. Pack into rigid containers, label, and freeze.

4. To thaw and reheat: Thaw overnight in refrigerator. Place beef and sauce in heavy skillet, cover, and bring to a boil over medium heat. Reduce heat and simmer for 10 to 14 minutes, until rolls are thoroughly hot in the center.

Burgundy Beef

This rich stew is delicious served over hot cooked egg noodles. To serve without freezing, simply serve stew after 2 to 3 hours of simmering.

Serves 6–8

2 onions, chopped

4 cloves garlic, chopped

3 tablespoons olive oil 2 pounds cubed beef ¼ cup flour

½ teaspoon salt 2 (4-ounce) cans sliced mushrooms

1 (6-ounce) can tomato paste

2 cups burgundy wine

3 cups Beef Broth

2 teaspoons dried thyme leaves

1 teaspoon pepper

1 (9-ounce) package baby carrots

Serves 18–24

6 onions, chopped

12 cloves garlic, chopped

9 tablespoons olive oil

6 pounds cubed beef

¾ cup flour

1½ teaspoons salt

6 (4-ounce) cans sliced mushrooms

3 (6-ounce) cans tomato paste

6 cups burgundy wine

9 cups Beef Broth

6 teaspoons dried thyme leaves

1 teaspoon pepper

3 (9-ounce) packages baby carrots

1. In heavy stockpot, sauté onions and garlic in olive oil until crisp-tender. Remove vegetables

from pan. On shallow plate, toss beef with flour and salt. Add beef to drippings in pan in

batches; sauté each batch 3 to 4 minutes, until browned.

2. Return onions and garlic to pan along with remaining ingredients, except carrots. Bring to a boil, then cover, reduce heat, and simmer for 2 to 3 hours, until beef is very tender.

3. Cool beef mixture in an ice-water bath or in refrigerator. Pack into 1-gallon-size zipper-lock bag;

attach bag with baby carrots; label, seal and freeze.

4. To thaw and reheat: Thaw beef mixture and carrots overnight in refrigerator. Pour beef mixture into saucepan and add carrots; bring to a boil, then reduce heat and simmer for 15 to 20 minutes until hot.

Mexican Quiche

This quiche is delicious topped with salsa and sour cream. To serve immediately, bake at 375°F for 40 to 45 minutes, until set and golden brown.

Serves 6

½ cup refried beans

1 9-inch Pie Crust

1 pound sirloin steak

1 onion, chopped

3 cloves garlic, chopped

2 tablespoons olive oil

1 (4-ounce) can chopped green chilies

1½ cups grated pepper jack cheese

4 eggs

½ cup sour cream

½ cup grated Parmesan cheese

Serves 18

1½ cups refried beans

3 9-inch Pie Crusts

3 pounds sirloin steak

3 onions, chopped

9 cloves garlic, chopped

6 tablespoons olive oil

3 (4-ounce) cans chopped green chilies

4½ cups grated pepper jack cheese

12 eggs

1½ cups sour cream

1½ cups grated Parmesan cheese

1. Preheat oven to 375°F. Spread refried beans in bottom of unbaked pie crust and set aside. Cut steak into ½-inch pieces. In heavy skillet, brown steak with onion and garlic in olive oil.

Remove from pan with slotted spoon and place in pie crust. Sprinkle drained green chilies overall. Sprinkle pepper jack cheese over green chilies.

2. In medium bowl, combine eggs and sour cream and beat to mix well. Pour over cheese in pie crust; sprinkle Parmesan cheese on top. Bake at 375°F for 35 to 40 minutes until quiche is set and top is light golden brown. Cool in refrigerator; then wrap in freezer wrap, label, and freeze.

Or, slice cooled quiche into slices before freezing and flash freeze individually.

3. To thaw and reheat: Thaw quiche overnight in refrigerator. Bake at 350°F for 20 to 25 minutes
until heated through.

To reheat individual slices: Microwave each frozen slice on medium power for 2 to 4 minutes, then 1 minute on high.

Curried Beef Stew

To serve this stew immediately, just add the frozen potatoes and peas to simmering stew and cook over medium heat, stirring occasionally, for 75 to 25 minutes, until vegetables are hot and tender.

Serves 4–6

1 onion, chopped

2 shallots, minced

2 tablespoons olive oil

1 pound chuck steak

3 tablespoons flour

2 teaspoons curry powder

1 teaspoon salt

4 cups Beef Broth

1½ cups frozen potato wedges

1 cup frozen baby peas

2 cups baby carrots

Serves 12–18

3 onions, chopped

6 shallots, minced

6 tablespoons olive oil

3 pounds chuck steak

9 tablespoons flour

6 teaspoons curry powder

1 tablespoon salt

12 cups Beef Broth

4½ cups frozen potato wedges

3 cups frozen baby peas 6 cups baby carrots

1. Cook onion and shallots in olive oil until crisp-tender, stirring frequently. Remove vegetables from pan with slotted spoon. Cut chuck steak into 1-inch pieces. Combine flour, curry powder, and salt in a shallow plate and toss steak cubes to coat.

2. Brown steak in drippings remaining in pan for 3 to 4 minutes, stirring occasionally. Return onion and shallots to pan and add beef broth. Bring to a boil, then cover pan, reduce heat, and simmer for 1½ hours until beef is tender.

3. Cool stew in ice-water bath or in refrigerator. Pour stew into gallon-size zipper-lock bags and place frozen potato wedges and peas in quart zipper-lock bag; attach to stew. Attach bag with baby carrots; then label and freeze.

4. To thaw and reheat: Thaw stew and carrots overnight in refrigerator. Keep potatoes and peas frozen. Pour stew and carrots into large saucepan and bring to a boil over medium-high heat.

Reduce heat, add frozen potatoes and peas, and simmer for 15 to 25 minutes until stew is hot and potatoes are tender.

Marinated Round Steak

To serve without freezing, let meat marinate 4 to 8 hours, or overnight, in the refrigerator. Then grill or broil steak, turning once, until desired doneness.

Serves 4–6

2 pounds bottom round steak

1 cup red wine vinegar

3 tablespoons olive oil

3 cloves garlic, minced

½ teaspoon salt

1 teaspoon pepper

1 teaspoon dried thyme leaves

2 tablespoons sugar

½ teaspoon celery salt

Serves 12–18

3 (2-pound) bottom round steaks

1 cup red wine vinegar

9 tablespoons olive oil

9 cloves garlic, minced

1½ teaspoons salt

1 teaspoon pepper

1 tablespoon dried thyme leaves

6 tablespoons sugar

1½ teaspoons celery salt

1. Trim excess fat off steak and cut into 4 to 6 serving pieces. Pierce steak with fork in several places.

2. In gallon zipper-lock bag, combine remaining ingredients to make marinade. Add steak; then seal and massage bag to work the marinade into the meat. Label bag and freeze.

3. To thaw and cook: Thaw meat overnight in the refrigerator. Grill or broil steak for 10 to 20 minutes, turning once, until desired doneness. Let meat stand, covered, for 10 minutes before slicing.

Phyllo Chicken Roll

This elegant entree is perfect for a brunch. To serve immediately, bake roll at 375°F for 40 to 50 minutes, until pastry is crisp and golden brown and filling is thoroughly heated.

Serves 4

1 red bell pepper, chopped

1 onion, chopped

2 cloves garlic, minced

1 cup chopped mushrooms

1 tablespoon olive oil

½ cup ricotta cheese

1 egg

1 cup shredded Gruyère cheese

¼ cup grated Parmesan cheese

2 cups cooked, cubed chicken breast

6 sheets thawed phyllo dough

¼ cup melted butter

Serves 12

3 red bell peppers, chopped

3 onions, chopped

6 cloves garlic, minced

3 cups chopped mushrooms

3 tablespoons olive oil

1½ cups ricotta cheese

3 eggs

3 cups shredded Gruyère cheese

¾ A cup grated Parmesan cheese

6 cups cooked, cubed chicken breast

18 sheets thawed phyllo dough

¾ A cup melted butter

1. In large skillet, sauté bell pepper, onion, garlic, and mushrooms in olive oil until crisp-tender, stirring frequently. Let cool for 20 minutes.

2. In large bowl, combine ricotta cheese and egg and beat until combined. Add Gruyère, Parmesan, and cooked chicken and mix well. Stir in cooled vegetable mixture until well blended.

3. Place one sheet phyllo dough on the large cookie sheet and brush with butter. Top with the remaining five sheets, brushing each lightly with butter. Place chicken mixture along one edge of the dough, leaving a 1-inch margin. Fold in short ends of phyllo dough,

and then roll, starting with side containing filling. Seal edges with butter. Brush the entire roll with remaining melted butter. Wrap roll in foil, label, and freeze.

4. To thaw and cook: Partially unwrap and thaw chicken roll overnight in refrigerator. Brush with 1 tablespoon melted butter. Bake in preheated 375°F oven for 40 to 50 minutes until the pastry is crisp and golden brown and filling is thoroughly heated. Let stand 10 minutes before serving.

Slice carefully on the diagonal using a serrated knife.

Chicken Fried Rice

To serve immediately, stir-fry the rice mixture in olive oil until hot. Beat eggs and add to skillet. Cook eggs until set but still moist. Add soy sauce and sesame oil and serve.

Serves 4

1½ cups long-grain white rice

2½ cups water

1 onion, chopped

1 cup frozen soybeans

2 cups cooked, cubed chicken breast

2 tablespoons olive oil

2 tablespoons soy sauce

1 teaspoon toasted sesame oil

3 eggs

½ teaspoon salt

1 teaspoon pepper

Serves 12

4½ cups long-grain white rice

7½ cups water

3 onions, chopped

3 cups frozen soybeans

6 cups cooked, cubed chicken breast

6 tablespoons olive oil

6 tablespoons soy sauce

1 tablespoon toasted sesame oil

9 eggs

1½ teaspoons salt

1 teaspoon pepper

1. Combine rice and water in heavy saucepan. Bring to boil over high heat. Reduce heat to low, cover pan, and cook rice until almost tender but still firm in the center, about 15 minutes. Gently fluff rice with fork. Spread rice into a thin layer on a foil-lined cookie sheet and refrigerate until very cold.

2. Gently break up clumps of rice and mix with chopped onions, frozen soybeans, and cooked cubed chicken. Package in zipper-lock bag, label, and freeze.

3. Mark olive oil, soy sauce, and toasted sesame oil as reserved ingredients and store in your pantry. Mark eggs as reserved in refrigerator.

4. To thaw and cook: Let rice mixture thaw overnight in refrigerator. Heat olive oil in large skillet or wok. Stir-fry rice mixture in oil until thoroughly heated. Push rice mixture to one side of wok and pour in beaten eggs. Stir-fry until eggs are set but still moist. Gently stir the set eggs into rice/chicken mixture. Season with soy sauce, sesame oil, salt, and pepper, and serve immediately.

Chicken Tucson

This easy casserole takes about 10 minutes to assemble. To serve immediately, dollop with sour cream and sprinkle with cheese. Bake at 350°F for 25 to 35 minutes until bubbly and cheese begins to brown.

Serves 4

1 (20-ounce) jar salsa

2 (16-ounce) cans black beans

1 red bell pepper, chopped

2 cups cooked, cubed chicken breast

6 corn tortillas

2 cups shredded Cheddar cheese

½ cup sour cream

Serves 12

3 (20-ounce) jars salsa

6 (16-ounce) cans black beans

3 red bell peppers, chopped

6 cups cooked, cubed chicken breast

18 corn tortillas

6 cups shredded Cheddar cheese

1½ cups sour cream

1. Spread ½ cup salsa in 9″ × 9″ baking dish and set aside. Drain black beans and rinse well; drain again. In large bowl, combine beans, bell pepper, chicken, and remaining salsa and mix well.

2. Place 3 tortillas on salsa at the bottom of the baking dish. Top with half of chicken mixture and sprinkle with half of cheese. Top with 3 more tortillas, then remaining chicken mixture. Wrap and label. Reserve sour cream in refrigerator. Place remaining cheese in zipper-lock bag, attach to the baking dish and freeze.

3. To thaw and cook: Thaw overnight in the refrigerator. Place small dollops of sour cream on casserole and top with reserved cheese. Bake at 350°F for 30 to 40 minutes until hot and cheese begins to brown.

Cheesy Chicken Manicotti

To serve immediately, sprinkle casserole with cheese and bake at 350°F for 80 to 90 minutes, until chicken is cooked and casserole is bubbly.

Serves 6

1 teaspoon Italian seasoning

2 cloves garlic, minced

¼ cup grated Parmesan cheese

1½ pounds chicken tenders

14 manicotti shells

1 (26-ounce) jar tomato pasta sauce

2 cups frozen peppers and onions

½ cup of water

1 (14-ounce) jar Alfredo sauce

½ cup Parmesan cheese

1 cup shredded mozzarella cheese

Serves 18

1 tablespoon Italian seasoning

6 cloves garlic, minced

¾ cup grated Parmesan cheese

4½ pounds chicken tenders

42 manicotti shells

3 (26-ounce) jars tomato pasta sauce

6 cups frozen peppers and onions

1½ cups water

3 (14-ounce) jars Alfredo sauce

1½ cups Parmesan cheese

3 cups shredded mozzarella cheese

1. In shallow bowl, combine Italian seasoning, minced garlic, and first quantity grated Parmesan cheese. Toss chicken tenders with this mixture until coated. Place one coated chicken tender inside each uncooked manicotti shell.

2. Pour 1 cup tomato pasta sauce inlined 13″ × 9″ baking dish. Arrange filled manicotti shells in dish. Arrange frozen bell peppers and onions around manicotti shells. Add water to remaining tomato pasta sauce in jar and mix well. Pour over vegetables and manicotti shells. Pour Alfredo sauce overall.

3. Freeze casserole until hard, then remove from dish and wrap again. In zipper-lock bag, combine remaining Parmesan cheese and mozzarella cheese. Attach to casserole, label, and freeze.

4. To thaw and cook: Thaw casserole overnight in refrigerator. Sprinkle with cheeses. Cover casserole with foil and bake at 350°F for 80 to 95 minutes until chicken is thoroughly cooked, pasta is tender, cheese is beginning to brown, and casserole is bubbly.

Sweet and Sour Chicken Stew

To serve immediately, mix cornstarch and water together and add to simmering stew. Cook 5 to 8 minutes longer, until slightly thickened.

Serves 4

3 boneless, skinless chicken breasts

1 onion, chopped

2 cloves garlic, chopped

2 tablespoons olive oil

1 (10-ounce) can pineapple chunks

¼ cup apple cider vinegar

¼ cup of sugar

3 cups Chicken Broth

1 red bell pepper, chopped

1 green bell pepper, chopped

2 tablespoons cornstarch

¼ cup of water

Serves 12

9 boneless, skinless chicken breasts

3 onions, chopped

6 cloves garlic, chopped

6 tablespoons olive oil

3 (10-ounce) cans pineapple chunks

¾ cup apple cider vinegar

¾ cup of sugar

9 cups Chicken Broth

3 red bell peppers, chopped

3 green bell peppers, chopped

6 tablespoons cornstarch

¾ cup of water

1. Cut chicken into 1-inch pieces. In heavy stockpot, sauté chicken, onion, and garlic in olive oil until vegetables are crisp-tender. Add undrained pineapple chunks, vinegar, sugar, and chicken broth and stir well. Simmer for 20 to 30 minutes, stirring occasionally, until chicken is thoroughly cooked.

2. Cool stew in ice-water bath or refrigerator until cold. Pour into rigid quart containers, label, and freeze. Attach bag with chopped green and red peppers. Reserve cornstarch in pantry.

3. To reheat: Place frozen chicken mixture in top of double boiler and add bell peppers. Reheat over simmering water, stirring occasionally, until hot. In small bowl, combine cornstarch and water and mix well. Add cornstarch mixture to double boiler and cook over medium heat, stirring frequently, until sauce is thickened.

Chicken Potato Skillet

To serve immediately, sauté chicken in olive oil, then add vegetables. Cook and stir until vegetables are hot. Add soup and milk, cover, and simmer for 10 minutes. Add cheese and serve.

Serves 4

2 boneless, skinless chicken breasts

2 cups frozen potato wedges

1 cup frozen green beans

1 onion, chopped

1 (10-ounce) can cream of chicken soup

½ cup milk

1 cup grated Swiss cheese

2 tablespoons olive oil

Serves 12

6 boneless, skinless chicken breasts

6 cups frozen potato wedges

3 cups frozen green beans

3 onions, chopped

3 (10-ounce) cans cream of chicken soup

1½ cups milk

3 cups grated Swiss cheese

6 tablespoons olive oil

1. Cut chicken breasts into 1-inch pieces and place them in a zipper-lock bag. Combine frozen potatoes, green beans, and chopped onion and place in another zipper-lock bag. Combine soup and milk in a small bowl and pour it into a third zipper-lock bag. Place grated cheese in a fourth zipper-lock bag. Place all bags inside a larger bag, label, and freeze. Reserve olive oil in the pantry.

2. To thaw and cook: Thaw overnight in the refrigerator. Heat 2 tablespoons olive oil in skillet and add chicken. Cook and stir for 5 minutes until almost done. Add thawed vegetables; cook and stir 10 to 15 minutes longer, until vegetables are hot and potatoes start to crisp. Add soup mixture and cover. Simmer 10 minutes until flavors are blended. Sprinkle with cheese and serve.

Fragrant Sticky Chicken

To serve this delicious chicken without freezing, cook marinated chicken over medium heat for 6 to 8 minutes, then add honey, cover skillet, and cook 7 to 9 minutes longer or until chicken is thoroughly cooked.

Serves 4

1 cup of soy sauce

½ cup Chicken Broth

1 tablespoon grated gingerroot

4 boneless, skinless chicken breasts

3 cloves garlic, minced

¼ cup honey

Serves 12

1 cup of soy sauce

1½ cups Chicken Broth

3 tablespoons grated ginger root

6 cloves garlic, minced

12 boneless, skinless chicken breasts

¾ cup honey

1. In medium bowl, combine soy sauce, broth, ginger root, and garlic. Mix well, then add chicken breasts. Cover and marinate for 1 to 2 hours in the refrigerator; then pack into zipper-lock bag, label, and freeze. Reserve honey in the pantry.

2. To thaw and cook: Thaw chicken in marinade overnight in the refrigerator. Heat 12-inch skillet over medium heat, then add chicken and marinade. Cook 5 to 8 minutes on one side, then turn chicken, add honey, cover, and cook an additional 8 to 10 minutes until chicken is thoroughly cooked and sauce is reduced.

Chicken Santa Fe Soup

To serve immediately, garnish soup with tortilla chips, sour cream, salsa, or chopped tomatoes. Serve with a simple fruit salad and some cornbread.

Serves 4

2 boneless, skinless chicken breasts

1 onion, chopped

2 tablespoons olive oil

1 (16-ounce) can black beans, drained

1 (4-ounce) can green chilies, drained

1 teaspoon red pepper flakes

1 (16-ounce) can corn, drained

3 cups Chicken Broth

Serves 12

6 boneless, skinless chicken breasts

3 onions, chopped

6 tablespoons olive oil

3 (16-ounce) cans black beans, drained

3 (4-ounce) cans green chilies, drained

teaspoon red pepper flakes

3 (16-ounce) cans corn, drained

9 cups Chicken Broth

1. Cut chicken breasts into 1-inch pieces. In heavy skillet, sauté chicken and onion in olive oil until onion is crisp-tender. Add remaining ingredients, stir to blend, and simmer for 10 to 15 minutes. Cool soup in refrigerator or ice bath. Pour soup into rigid containers; seal, label, and freeze.

2. To thaw and reheat: Thaw soup overnight in the refrigerator, then reheat in heavy saucepan until bubbling.

To reheat from frozen: Place frozen soup in top of double boiler; heat over simmering water, stirring occasionally, until soup is hot. Transfer to saucepan and heat until bubbling.

Citrus Glazed Chicken

To serve immediately, marinate chicken in the refrigerator for up to 6 hours. Bake at 350°F for 25 to 30 minutes, until chicken is thoroughly cooked, basting frequently.

Serves 4

4 boneless, skinless chicken breasts

¼ cup honey

3 tablespoons lemon juice

2 tablespoons orange juice

1 teaspoon dried tarragon

Serves 12

12 boneless, skinless chicken breasts

¾ cup honey

9 tablespoons lemon juice

6 tablespoons orange juice

1 tablespoon dried tarragon

1. Place chicken in a zipper-lock bag. Mix remaining ingredients in medium bowl to make marinade and pour over chicken. Seal bag, label, and freeze.

2. To thaw and reheat: Thaw chicken overnight in refrigerator. Uncover and bake chicken at 350°F for 25 to 30 minutes, basting frequently, until chicken is thoroughly cooked and glazed.

Creamy Bacon Chicken

To serve immediately, crumble bacon and sprinkle over casserole. Sprinkle cheese over bacon. Bake at 350°F for 18 to 25 minutes, until chicken is thoroughly cooked and cheese is melted.

Serves 4

5 slices bacon

8 ounces mushrooms, chopped

4 boneless, skinless chicken breasts

1 (10-ounce) jar Alfredo sauce

1 cup grated Havarti cheese

Serves 12

5 slices bacon

3 (8-ounce) packages mushrooms, chopped

12 boneless, skinless chicken breasts

3 (10-ounce) jars Alfredo sauce

3 cups grated Havarti cheese

1. In heavy skillet, cook bacon until crisp. Remove bacon from pan and drain on paper towels. Sauté mushrooms in bacon drippings. Place uncooked chicken in 9″ × 9″ baking dish; top with mushrooms. Pour Alfredo sauce overall. Cool in refrigerator, then wrap, attach bag with bacon and another bag with cheese, label, and freeze.

2. To thaw and reheat: Thaw casserole overnight in refrigerator. Crumble bacon and sprinkle over all. Sprinkle cheese over bacon. Bake at 375°F for 20 to 25 minutes, until thoroughly heated and chicken is thoroughly cooked.

Chicken Risotto

To serve immediately, continue cooking rice mixture, adding 1 cup water and condensed chicken broth until rice is tender and chicken is cooked through. Add remaining ingredients and cook until hot.

Serves 4

3 boneless, skinless chicken breasts

2 tablespoons olive oil

1 onion, chopped

1 cup chopped leeks

2 cups long-grain white rice

1 cup white wine

1 cup Chicken Broth

½ cup grated Parmesan cheese

1 (10-ounce) can condensed chicken broth

3 tablespoons heavy cream

3 tablespoons butter

Serves 12

9 boneless, skinless chicken breasts

6 tablespoons olive oil

3 onions, chopped

1½ cups chopped leeks

6 cups long-grain white rice

3 cups white wine

3 cups Chicken Broth

1½ cups grated Parmesan cheese

3 (10-ounce) cans condensed chicken broth

9 tablespoons heavy cream

9 tablespoons butter

1. Cut chicken breasts into 1-inch pieces. Heat olive oil in large stockpot. Add chicken, onion, and leeks; cook and stir for 5 to 7 minutes until onion is crisp-tender and chicken turns white.

2. Add uncooked rice and stir well until rice is coated. Cook for 2 to 3 minutes over medium heat, until rice begins to look translucent. Add white wine and cook, stirring frequently, until liquid is absorbed. Turn heat down to low; add plain chicken broth and cook, stirring frequently, until liquid is absorbed.

3. Remove pan from heat and place mixture in rigid containers. Chill in refrigerator or ice-water bath; then wrap, pack, and freeze. Attach bag with grated cheese. Reserve condensed chicken broth in pantry, and cream and butter in the fridge.

4. To thaw and reheat: Thaw overnight in refrigerator. Place in saucepan over low heat, stirring occasionally, until hot. Combine reserved condensed chicken broth with 1 cup water and add to rice mixture. Cook and stir over medium heat until liquid is absorbed, rice is tender, and chicken is cooked through. Add cheese, cream, and butter, and stir until cheese and butter are melted.

Chicken Divan Soup

To serve immediately, add broccoli to soup when chicken is cooked through. Cook for 4 to 5 minutes longer, until broccoli is hot. Add grated cheese; cook and stir until cheese melts, about 3 to 4 minutes.

Serves 4

2 boneless, skinless chicken breasts

1 onion, chopped

2 cloves garlic, chopped

2 tablespoons olive oil

3 cups Chicken Broth

1 teaspoon pepper

1 (10-ounce) can condensed broccoli cheese soup

1 (10-ounce) package frozen chopped broccoli

1 cup grated Swiss cheese

Serves 12

6 boneless, skinless chicken breasts

3 onions, chopped

6 cloves garlic, chopped

6 tablespoons olive oil

9 cups Chicken Broth

1 teaspoon pepper

3 (10-ounce) cans condensed broccoli cheese soup

3 (10-ounce) packages frozen chopped broccoli

3 cups grated Swiss cheese

1. Cut chicken breasts into 1-inch pieces. In large saucepan, cook chicken, onion, and garlic in olive oil until vegetables are crisp-tender. Add broth, pepper, and condensed soup; stir well. Simmer for 10 to 15 minutes, until chicken is thoroughly cooked.

2. Chill soup in an ice-water bath or refrigerator. Place in rigid containers and attach a package of frozen broccoli and bag of grated cheese. Wrap, label, and freeze.

3. To thaw and reheat: Thaw everything overnight in refrigerator. Place soup and broccoli in saucepan and heat over medium-low heat until soup simmers. Add cheese and stir for 2 to 3 minutes, until cheese melts.

Cheesy Chicken Supreme

To serve immediately, don't refrigerate. Add crumbled bacon and cheese to skillet; cover and cook over medium-low heat for 4 to 5 minutes, until cheese is melted and mixture is bubbly. Serve over hot cooked couscous.

Serves 4

4 slices bacon

4 boneless, skinless chicken breasts

1 onion, chopped

2 cloves garlic, chopped

1 (10-ounce) can condensed mushroom soup

½ cup milk

1 cup grated Havarti cheese

1 (6-ounce) package couscous

Serves 14

12 slices bacon

12 boneless, skinless chicken breasts

3 onions, chopped

6 cloves garlic, chopped

3 (10-ounce) cans condensed mushroom soup

1½ cups milk

3 cups grated Havarti cheese

3 (6-ounce) packages couscous

1. In large skillet, cook bacon until crisp; remove from pan and drain on paper towels. Add chicken to drippings remaining in skillet; cook 2 to 3 minutes on each side.

2. Add onion and garlic to skillet; cook and stir for 4 to 5 minutes, until crisp-tender. Add soup and milk; stir to blend. Simmer until chicken is thoroughly cooked. Chill chicken mixture in refrigerator or ice-water bath.

3. Crumble bacon and place in zipper-lock bag. Place cheese in a zipper-lock bag. Place chilled chicken and sauce in a zipper-lock bag. Place all bags inside a larger bag; label and freeze. Reserve couscous in pantry.

4. To thaw and reheat: Thaw overnight in refrigerator. Place chicken mixture in skillet and heat for about 10 minutes, until hot. Add bacon and cheese to skillet; cover and cook on low heat for 5 to 6 minutes, until chicken is thoroughly heated. Serve over hot cooked couscous.

Lemon Chicken

To serve immediately, mix cornstarch with water and add to simmering sauce. Cook for 3 to 4 minutes, until thickened. Drain mandarin oranges and add; cook 2 to 3 minutes, until hot.

Serves 4

4 boneless, skinless chicken breasts

2 cloves garlic, chopped

2 tablespoons olive oil

½ cup orange juice

¼ cup lemon juice

2 teaspoons grated lemon peel

½ cup Chicken Broth

½ teaspoon salt

1 teaspoon pepper

2 tablespoons cornstarch

1 (16-ounce) can mandarin oranges

¼ cup of water

Serves 12

12 boneless, skinless chicken breasts

6 cloves garlic, chopped

6 tablespoons olive oil

1½ cups orange juice

¾ cup lemon juice

2 tablespoons grated lemon peel

1½ cups Chicken Broth

1½ teaspoons salt

teaspoon pepper

6 tablespoons cornstarch

3 (16-ounce) cans mandarin oranges

¾ cup of water

1. Cut chicken breasts in half crosswise. Cook chicken and garlic in olive oil until chicken is browned on both sides. Add orange juice,

lemon juice and peel, broth, salt, and pepper to skillet. Simmer until chicken is thoroughly cooked, about 10 to 12 minutes.

2. Pour chicken and sauce into rigid containers and cool in refrigerator. Reserve cornstarch and mandarin oranges in the pantry. Wrap chicken, label, and freeze.

3. To thaw and reheat: Thaw overnight in refrigerator. Pour chicken and sauce into a heavy saucepan and bring to a simmer. Mix cornstarch and water in small bowl and add to saucepan.

Cook and stir until thickened, 3 to 4 minutes. Drain mandarin oranges and add to skillet; simmer until heated through. Serve over hot cooked rice.

Orange Curried Chicken

Serve this delicious Indian dish with extra curry powder for those who like it hot. To serve immediately, add frozen peppers and onions and simmer 5 to 8 minutes until hot; serve over rice.

Serves 4

4 boneless, skinless chicken breasts

3 tablespoons flour

1 tablespoon curry powder

1 teaspoon salt

3 tablespoons olive oil

1 cup of orange juice

½ cup evaporated milk

2 cups frozen peppers and onions

Serves 12

12 boneless, skinless chicken breasts

9 tablespoons flour

3 tablespoons curry powder

1 tablespoon salt

9 tablespoons olive oil

3 cups orange juice

1½ cups evaporated milk

6 cups frozen peppers and onions

1. Cut chicken breasts into 1-inch pieces. Combine flour, curry powder, and salt in a large plate. Add chicken and toss to coat.

2. Heat olive oil in large skillet. Add chicken; cook and stir until chicken is almost cooked. Add orange juice; simmer for 10 to 15 minutes, until chicken is thoroughly cooked. Add evaporated milk, stir, and remove from heat.

3. Chill mixture in refrigerator or ice-water bath until cold. Add frozen vegetables and mix gently. Wrap, label, and freeze.

4. To thaw and reheat: Thaw mixture overnight in refrigerator. Place in heavy skillet and cook over medium heat for 10 to 15 minutes, until bubbly and thoroughly heated. Serve over hot cooked rice.

Chicken on Cornbread

To serve immediately, bake the cornbread at 400°F for 20 to 25 minutes until golden brown around edges. Heat chicken in gravy and pour over squares of hot cornbread.

Serves 4

½ cup flour

½ cup yellow cornmeal

¼ teaspoon baking soda

½ teaspoon baking powder

½ teaspoon salt

2 tablespoons chopped green chilies

3 tablespoons vegetable oil

½ cup buttermilk

1 egg, beaten

¼ cup minced onion

¼ cup butter

¼ cup flour

½ teaspoon salt

1 teaspoon pepper

1 cup Chicken Broth

½ cup milk

2 cooked chicken breasts

Serves 12

1½ cups flour

1½ cups yellow cornmeal

¾ teaspoons baking soda

1½ teaspoons baking powder

1 teaspoon salt

6 tablespoons chopped green chilies

9 tablespoons vegetable oil

1½ cups buttermilk

3 eggs, beaten

¾ cup minced onion

¾ cup butter

¾ cup flour

1 teaspoon salt

1 teaspoon pepper

3 cups Chicken Broth

1½ cups milk

6 cooked chicken breasts

1. Preheat oven to 400°F. Line 8″ × 8″ pan with foil and grease. In large bowl, combine flour, cornmeal, baking soda, baking powder, and salt. In small bowl, combine green chilies, oil, buttermilk, and egg. Mix with dry ingredients. Pour mixture into prepared pan and bake at 400°F for 15 minutes, until set; cool.

2. Meanwhile, in large saucepan, cook onion in butter for 3 to 4 minutes. Add flour, salt, and pepper; cook and stir 2 to 3 minutes. Add broth and milk; cook and stir 5 to 6 minutes. Cool gravy in an ice-water bath or refrigerator.

3. Remove baked cornbread from pan and wrap again in foil. Slice chicken and put in 1-quart zipper-lock bag with gravy. Seal bag, attach to cornbread, then label and freeze.

4. To thaw and reheat: Thaw cornbread and chicken overnight in refrigerator. Unwrap cornbread and place in pan; bake at 400°F for 8 to 10 minutes or until hot and golden. Place chicken and gravy in the skillet and cook over low heat for 8 to 11 minutes or until hot. Serve chicken and gravy over hot cornbread squares.

Grandma's Chicken Soup

To serve immediately, simmer carrots and frozen vegetables in broth for 5 minutes. Add chicken and egg noodles and simmer 4 to 5 minutes longer, until noodles and vegetables are tender.

Serves 6–8

3-pound stewing chicken, cut up

1 teaspoon salt

1 teaspoon pepper

2 tablespoons olive oil

1 onion, chopped

4 cloves garlic, chopped

5 cups of water

3 carrots, sliced

2 cups frozen pearl onions

1 cup frozen peas

1 cup frozen green beans

1 cup uncooked egg noodles

Serves 18–24

3 (3-pound) stewing chickens, cut up

1 tablespoon salt

1 teaspoon pepper

6 tablespoons olive oil

3 onions, chopped

12 cloves garlic, chopped

15 cups water

9 carrots, sliced

6 cups frozen pearl onions

3 cups frozen peas

3 cups frozen green beans

3 cups uncooked egg noodles

1. Sprinkle chicken with salt and pepper and set aside. Heat olive oil in large stockpot or Dutch oven over medium heat and sauté onion and garlic until crisp-tender. Add chicken pieces and water to pot. Bring to a boil; then cover, reduce heat, and simmer for 70 to 80 minutes, until chicken is thoroughly cooked. Remove chicken from broth, remove and discard skin and bones; strain broth. Wash stockpot and dry thoroughly.

2. Place broth in stockpot and add carrots. Simmer for 5 to 7 minutes, until carrots are tender. Add chicken meat and cool soup in an ice-water bath or in refrigerator. Stir in pearl onions, peas, and

green beans. Pour soup into rigid containers, label, and freeze. Reserve egg noodles in the pantry.

3. To thaw and reheat: Thaw soup in refrigerator overnight. Place in a large stockpot or Dutch oven. Bring to a simmer over medium heat, stirring occasionally. Add egg noodles and cook for 4 to 5 minutes, until tender.

Spanish Chicken and Olives

To serve immediately, bake until chicken pieces are tender, removing cover for last 10 minutes of cooking time. Serve with hot cooked rice or mashed potatoes.

Serves 6–8

2 pounds chicken pieces

1 teaspoon salt

1 teaspoon pepper

1 teaspoon paprika

2 tablespoons olive oil

5 cloves garlic, chopped

1 (14-ounce) can diced tomatoes, undrained

1 (6-ounce) can tomato paste

1 cup Chicken Broth

1 cup sliced pimento-stuffed olives

Serves 18–24

6 pounds chicken pieces

1 tablespoon salt

1 teaspoon pepper

1 tablespoon paprika

6 tablespoons olive oil

15 cloves garlic, chopped

3 (14-ounce) cans diced tomatoes, undrained

3 (6-ounce) cans tomato paste

3 cups Chicken Broth

3 cups sliced pimento-stuffed olives

1. Sprinkle chicken pieces with salt, pepper, and paprika. Heat olive oil in large skillet. Add chicken in batches, skin-side down. Sauté until skin browns, turning once, about 5–8 minutes. Remove chicken from pan as it browns.

2. When all the chicken is browned, add garlic, diced tomatoes, tomato paste, and broth to skillet. Bring to a boil, scraping up pan drippings.

3. Preheat oven to 350°F. Place chicken in 9" × 13" baking dish. Pour mixture in skillet over chicken. Sprinkle with olives, cover, and bake at 350°F for 60 to 70 minutes, until chicken is tender and thoroughly cooked. Cool in ice-water bath or refrigerator. Place in zipper-lock bags, seal, label, and freeze.

4. To thaw and reheat: Thaw in refrigerator overnight. Place mixture in heavy skillet. Bring to a boil, reduce heat, and simmer for 10 to 15 minutes, until chicken is thoroughly heated.

Spicy Thai Chicken

To serve this dish without freezing, marinate chicken for 3 to 4 hours in refrigerator. Cook chicken mixture in olive oil for 8 to 10 minutes, then add frozen vegetables; cook 5 to 8 minutes longer, until done.

Serves 4–6

½ cup orange juice

1 cup chunky peanut butter

½ teaspoon crushed red pepper

¼ teaspoon ground cumin

1 tablespoon curry powder

2 pounds boned, skinned chicken thighs

2 cups frozen peppers and onions

2 tablespoons olive oil

1 (6-ounce) package garlic couscous

Serves 12–18

1½ cups orange juice

1 cup chunky peanut butter

1½ teaspoons crushed red pepper

¾ A teaspoon ground cumin

3 tablespoons curry powder

6 pounds boned, skinned chicken thighs

6 cups frozen peppers and onions

6 tablespoons olive oil

3 (6-ounce) packages garlic couscous

1. Combine orange juice, peanut butter, and spices in a large zipper-lock bag. Cut chicken into 1- inch-wide strips and add to bag; mix by kneading the bag. Attach bag with frozen peppers and onions and place in larger bags. Label chicken and freeze. Reserve olive oil and couscous in pantry.

2. To thaw and reheat: Thaw all bags overnight in refrigerator. Heat olive oil in large skillet and add chicken mixture. Cook over medium-high heat, stirring frequently, for 8 to 10 minutes, until chicken is almost cooked. Drain peppers and onions and add to chicken in skillet. Cook and stir 3 to 6 minutes longer, until vegetables are hot and chicken is thoroughly cooked. Serve over prepared couscous.

Chicken Potato Pie

Hash brown potatoes form a crust in this delicious main-dish pie. To serve immediately, bake as directed. Let the pie stand 10 minutes before slicing.

Serves 6

For crust:

½ cup finely chopped onion

1 tablespoon olive oil

2 cups frozen hash brown potatoes, thawed

1 egg

For filling:

3 cups cooked, cubed chicken

1 cup frozen peas, thawed

1 cup shredded Gouda cheese

3 eggs

½ cup evaporated milk

½ teaspoon dried marjoram

½ teaspoon salt

1 teaspoon white pepper

Serves 18

For crust:

1½ cups finely chopped onion

3 tablespoons olive oil

6 cups frozen hash brown potatoes, thawed

3 eggs

For filling:

9 cups cooked, cubed chicken

3 cups frozen peas, thawed

3 cups shredded Gouda cheese

9 eggs

1½ cups evaporated milk

1½ teaspoons dried marjoram

1½ teaspoons salt

1 teaspoon white pepper

1. Preheat oven to 375°F. In heavy skillet, sauté onion in olive oil until tender. Remove from heat. Drain potatoes very well and add to

skillet along with a first egg. Mix well and press into a well-greased 9-inch pie pan. Bake at 375°F for 15 to 20 minutes, until crust begins to brown.

2. Place chicken and peas in potato crust and sprinkle with cheese. In medium bowl, beat eggs, milk, marjoram, salt, and pepper until blended. Pour egg mixture over cheese. Bake at 375°F for 25 to 35 minutes, until filling is puffed and set. Run knife around edge of pie pan to loosen crust.

Cool pie in refrigerator until cold, then wrap, label, and freeze.

3. To thaw and reheat: Thaw pie overnight in refrigerator. Bake at 375°F, uncovered, for 20 to 25 minutes, until thoroughly heated.

Chicken Cassoulet

To serve immediately, sprinkle casserole with the bread crumbs and bake at 375°F for 40 to 50 minutes, until bread crumbs are golden brown and casserole is bubbly.

Serves 4–6

2 cups dried Great Northern beans

½ pound sweet Italian pork sausage

2 tablespoons olive oil

1 onion, chopped

3 cloves garlic, chopped

1 cup chopped fennel

2 cups baby carrots

1 cup soft bread crumbs

2 tablespoons olive oil

2 cups cooked, cubed chicken

1 (14-ounce) can diced tomatoes, undrained

1 (10-ounce) can ready-to-serve chicken broth

1 teaspoon dried thyme leaves

Serves 12–18

6 cups dried Great Northern beans

1½ pounds sweet Italian pork sausage

6 tablespoons olive oil

3 onions, chopped

9 cloves garlic, chopped

3 cups chopped fennel

6 cups baby carrots

3 cups soft bread crumbs

6 tablespoons olive oil

6 cups cooked, cubed chicken

3 (14-ounce) cans diced tomatoes, undrained

3 (10-ounce) cans ready-to-serve chicken broth

1 tablespoon dried thyme leaves

1. In large stockpot, cover dried beans with water and bring to a boil. Boil for 1 minute, and then remove from heat, cover, and let stand for 1 hour. (Or place beans and 4 cups water in 4-quart slow cooker. Cover and cook on low for 8–10 hours, until beans are tender.) When cooked, drain and set aside.

2. Cut sausages into 1-inch slices. In large skillet, heat olive oil. Add sausages and cook, turning frequently, until browned. Remove from pan to large bowl. In drippings remaining in pan, sauté onion, garlic, and fennel until crisp-tender and remove from pan. Cut baby carrots in half lengthwise.

3. Combine bread crumbs and olive oil in a small zipper-lock bag. Combine all other ingredients in a large bowl and mix gently. Put meat-and-vegetable mixture in lined 3-quart baking dish. Cool in refrigerator, then wrap. Attach bag of bread crumb mixture to casserole, label, and freeze.

4. To thaw and reheat: Thaw casserole in refrigerator overnight. Sprinkle with bread crumbs and bake at 375°F for 45 to 55 minutes until golden brown and casserole is bubbly.

To heat from frozen: Cover casserole and bake at 375°F for 1 hour. Sprinkle with bread crumb mixture and bake another 25 to 35 minutes until bread crumbs are golden brown.

Lasagna Chicken Rolls

To serve this dish immediately, sprinkle reserved cheese over casserole and bake at 350°F for 40 to 45 minutes, until bubbly and cheese is golden brown.

Serves 6

1 onion, chopped

1 tablespoon olive oil

1 cup ricotta cheese

1 (3-ounce) package cream cheese

1 egg

1 cup shredded mozzarella cheese

½ cup grated Parmesan cheese

1 tablespoon cornstarch

2 cups cooked, cubed chicken

1 teaspoon dried basil leaves

6 lasagna noodles

2 cups prepared pasta sauce

1 cup grated mozzarella cheese

¼ cup grated Parmesan cheese

Serves 18

3 onions, chopped

3 tablespoons olive oil

3 cups ricotta cheese

1 (8-ounce) package cream cheese

3 eggs

3 cups shredded mozzarella cheese

1½ cups grated Parmesan cheese

3 tablespoons cornstarch

6 cups cooked, cubed chicken

1 tablespoon dried basil leaves

18 lasagna noodles

6 cups prepared pasta sauce

3 cups grated mozzarella cheese

¾ cup grated Parmesan cheese

1. In heavy skillet, sauté onion in olive oil until tender. Remove from heat and cool for 15 minutes.

In medium bowl, combine ricotta cheese, cream cheese, egg, 1 cup shredded mozzarella cheese,

½ cup Parmesan cheese, and cornstarch. Mix well until blended and creamy, then stir in sautéed onion, along with chicken and basil leaves.

2. Cook lasagna noodles as directed on package until slightly undercooked. Drain and rinse with cool water. Place noodles in a single layer on kitchen towel. Spread each cooked noodle with chicken mixture. Roll up each noodle, starting at the short end.

3. Place ½ cup pasta sauce in bottom of 9″ × 9″ square baking dish. Place filled lasagna rolls over pasta sauce. Pour remaining sauce over all. Cool in refrigerator, then wrap, seal, and label.

Place 1 cup mozzarella cheese and ¼ cup Parmesan cheese in a small zipper-lock bag and attach to dish. Wrap and freeze.

4. To thaw and reheat: Thaw casserole in refrigerator overnight. Bake at 350°F for 30 to 40 minutes, until hot and bubbly. Sprinkle cheese over all and bake 5 to 10 minutes longer, until cheese begins to brown. Let stand 10 minutes before serving.

Tortellini Chicken Cacciatore

You can serve this dish immediately by adding frozen tortellini to chicken mixture in skillet when chicken is thoroughly cooked. Simmer until tortellini is hot and tender.

Serves 6–8

3 tablespoons flour

1 teaspoon paprika

1 teaspoon salt

1 teaspoon pepper

2 pounds skinned chicken thighs and drumsticks

¼ cup olive oil

1 onion, chopped

5 cloves garlic, chopped

½ cup chopped celery

1 (8-ounce) package mushrooms, sliced

2 (14-ounce) cans diced tomatoes, undrained

½ cup white wine

1½ cups Chicken Broth

½ cup sliced ripe olives

1 (9-ounce) package frozen chicken tortellini

Serves 18–24

9 tablespoons flour

1 tablespoon paprika

1 tablespoon salt

1 teaspoon pepper

6 pounds skinned chicken thighs and drumsticks

¾ cup olive oil

3 onions, chopped

15 cloves garlic, chopped

1½ cups chopped celery

3 (8-ounce) packages mushrooms, sliced

6 (14-ounce) cans diced tomatoes, undrained

1½ cups white wine

4½ cups Chicken Broth

1½ cups sliced ripe olives

3 (9-ounce) packages frozen chicken tortellini

1. Combine flour, paprika, salt, and pepper on a shallow plate. Coat chicken pieces in flour mixture and shake off excess. Heat olive oil over medium heat in large skillet and cook chicken pieces, in batches, until browned, about 5 to 6 minutes per batch.

2. As chicken is cooked, remove from pan. When all chicken is browned, add onion, garlic, celery, and mushrooms to drippings remaining in pan. Cook and stir for 4 to 5 minutes, until crisp-tender.

Return chicken to pan and add undrained tomatoes, wine, broth, and olives. Cover pan and simmer for 40 to 50 minutes or until chicken is thoroughly cooked.

3. Cool cacciatore in an ice-water bath or refrigerator. When cold, pack into a zipper-lock bag. Attach frozen tortellini to bag; then label and freeze.

4. To thaw and reheat: Thaw overnight in refrigerator. In large skillet, bring chicken mixture to boil, reduce heat, and simmer for 10 to 12 minutes, until hot. Add tortellini to skillet and stir to make sure pasta is covered with sauce. (Add more broth if necessary to make mixture soupy.)

Cover pan and simmer for 3 to 4 minutes, until tortellini is tender and chicken is hot.

Herb Roasted Chicken

To serve without freezing, put the herb-rubbed chicken in the refrigerator for 2 to 3 hours, then brown in skillet and roast as directed in the recipe.

Serves 6–8

4 pounds of chicken pieces

2 tablespoons finely minced fresh rosemary

2 tablespoons minced fresh marjoram leaves

3 cloves garlic, minced

2 teaspoons salt

1 teaspoon white pepper

3 tablespoons mayonnaise

½ cup Chicken Broth

2 tablespoons olive oil

Serves 18–24

12 pounds of chicken pieces

6 tablespoons finely minced fresh rosemary

6 tablespoons minced fresh marjoram leaves

9 cloves garlic, minced

2 tablespoons salt

1 teaspoon white pepper

9 tablespoons mayonnaise

1½ cups Chicken Broth

6 tablespoons olive oil

1. Gently loosen the skin from the flesh of the chicken. In small bowl, combine herbs, garlic, salt, pepper, and mayonnaise, and rub this mixture between the skin and flesh of the chicken. Smooth skin back over chicken pieces.

2. Flash freeze chicken in a single layer on the baking sheet. When frozen solid, pack in zipper-lock bags; attach small bag with chicken broth. Label chicken and freeze. Reserve olive oil in the pantry.

3. To thaw and cook: Thaw chicken overnight in refrigerator. Preheat oven to 400°F. Meanwhile, heat olive oil in ovenproof skillet over medium heat. Place chicken, skin-side down, in pan and brown for 4 to 5 minutes. Turn chicken over and pour chicken broth into skillet. Place skillet in preheated oven, and roast for 30 to 40 minutes until chicken is thoroughly cooked and tender, basting occasionally with pan juices.

Lemon Drumsticks

To serve immediately, marinate chicken for 2 to 3 hours in the refrigerator, then bake at 375°F for 35 to 40 minutes, until thoroughly cooked and tender.

Serves 6

2 pounds chicken drumsticks

3 cloves garlic, minced

¼ cup lemon juice

2 tablespoons olive oil

½ cup Chicken Broth

1 teaspoon salt

1 teaspoon white pepper

1 teaspoon dried basil

Serves 18

6 pounds chicken drumsticks

9 cloves garlic, minced

¾ cup lemon juice

6 tablespoons olive oil

1½ cups Chicken Broth

1 tablespoon salt

1 teaspoon white pepper

1 tablespoon dried basil

1. Place drumsticks in a 1-gallon zipper-lock freezer bag. In medium bowl, combine remaining ingredients and mix well. Pour over

drumsticks, seal bag, and shake gently until chicken is coated; label and freeze.

2. To thaw and reheat: Thaw overnight in refrigerator. Preheat oven to 375°F. Pour contents of bag into 13″ × 9″ baking dish. Bake at 375°F for 35 to 45 minutes, until drumsticks are thoroughly cooked, basting occasionally with sauce.

Turkey Meatballs and Couscous

These tender meatballs are low in fat and very delicious. To serve immediately, combine hot meatballs with sauce and place in >casserole. Bake at 350°F for 20 to 25 minutes, until bubbly.

Serves 4–6

1 pound ground turkey

½ cup soft bread crumbs

¼ teaspoon garlic powder

½ teaspoon salt

½ teaspoon dried thyme leaves

1 egg

¼ cup evaporated milk

2 tablespoons olive oil

1 tablespoon butter

½ cup Chicken Broth

1 (16-ounce) jar Alfredo sauce

½ cup evaporated milk

1 cup grated Swiss cheese

1 (6-ounce) package couscous

Serves 12–18

3 pounds ground turkey

1½ cups soft bread crumbs

¾ teaspoon garlic powder

1½ teaspoons salt

1½ teaspoons dried thyme leaves

3 eggs

¾ cup evaporated milk

6 tablespoons olive oil

3 tablespoons butter

1½ cups Chicken Broth

3 (16-ounce) jars Alfredo sauce

1½ cups evaporated milk

3 cups grated Swiss cheese

3 (6-ounce) packages couscous

1. In large bowl, combine turkey, bread crumbs, garlic powder, salt, thyme, egg, and evaporated milk and mix to blend. Form into about 24 (or 72) meatballs.

2. Heat olive oil and butter in large skillet and cook meatballs in batches, removing to plate as they brown. Drain off excess fat, and then add chicken broth, return meatballs to skillet, cover, and simmer for 15 minutes or until meatballs are thoroughly cooked.

3. Cool meatballs in the refrigerator. When cold, combine with Alfredo sauce, evaporated milk, and Swiss cheese in 2-quart casserole. Wrap casserole, seal, label, and freeze. Reserve couscous in pantry.

4. To thaw and reheat: Thaw casserole overnight in refrigerator. Bake at 350°F for 30 to 40 minutes, until casserole is bubbly and thoroughly heated. Cook couscous according to package directions and serve with casserole.

Veggie Turkey Pizza

To serve without freezing, sprinkle cheeses over pizza and bake as directed until the crust is crisp and cheeses are melted.

Serves 4

1 cup ricotta cheese

1 tablespoon chopped chives

½ cup grated Parmesan cheese

1 teaspoon dried basil leaves

1 prebaked Pizza Crust

2 cups cooked, cubed turkey

2 cups frozen peppers and onions

1 cup shredded mozzarella cheese

1 cup shredded Monterey jack cheese

Serves 12

3 cups ricotta cheese

3 tablespoons chopped chives

1½ cups grated Parmesan cheese

1 tablespoon dried basil leaves

3 prebaked Pizza Crusts

6 cups cooked, cubed turkey

6 cups frozen peppers and onions

3 cups shredded mozzarella cheese

3 cups shredded Monterey jack cheese

1. In small bowl, combine ricotta, chives, Parmesan, and basil. Spread over pizza crust and top with turkey and frozen peppers and onions. Sprinkle with mozzarella and jack cheeses. Wrap pizza in freezer wrap, label, and freeze.

2. To cook: Preheat oven to 400°F. Place frozen pizza on baking sheet and bake at 400°F for 18 to 25 minutes or until pizza is hot, the crust is crisp, and cheeses are melted and beginning to brown.

Turkey Spinach Casserole

To serve this casserole without freezing, combine Parmesan cheese and bread crumbs and sprinkle over turkey mixture. Bake at 375°F for 20 to 25 minutes, until casserole bubbles and cheese browns.

Serves 4–6

1 onion, chopped

2 cloves garlic, minced

1 cup sliced carrots

2 tablespoons olive oil

2 cups cooked, cubed turkey

1 (14-ounce) jar pasta sauce

2 cups frozen cut-leaf spinach, thawed

1 cup ricotta cheese

1 egg

1 cup grated mozzarella cheese

1 cup grated Parmesan cheese

¼ cup dried Italian bread crumbs

Serves 12–18

3 onions, chopped

6 cloves garlic, minced

3 cups sliced carrots

6 tablespoons olive oil

6 cups cooked, cubed turkey

3 (14-ounce) jars pasta sauce

6 cups frozen cut-leaf spinach, thawed

3 cups ricotta cheese

3 eggs

3 cups grated mozzarella cheese

3 cups grated Parmesan cheese

¾ cup dried Italian bread crumbs

1. In heavy skillet, sauté onion, garlic, and carrots in olive oil until crisp-tender. Add turkey and pasta sauce and simmer for 5 minutes.

2. Meanwhile, thoroughly drain spinach and combine with ricotta, egg, and mozzarella. Place spinach mixture in 2-quart casserole and top with turkey mixture. Cool in ice-water bath or refrigerator; then wrap, label, attach small bag with Parmesan cheese and bread crumbs, and freeze.

3. To thaw and reheat: Thaw casserole overnight in refrigerator. Sprinkle with Parmesan cheese and bread crumb mixture and bake in preheated 375°F oven for 30 to 40 minutes, until bubbly and thoroughly heated.

Apricot Turkey Steaks

The apricot sauce is delicious served over hot noodles or rice. To serve without freezing, add apricot preserves to skillet during the last 3 to 4 minutes of cooking time and simmer until steaks are glazed.

Serves 4

4 turkey steaks

3 tablespoons flour

½ teaspoon salt

½ teaspoon cumin

3 tablespoons olive oil

1 cup apricot nectar

½ cup chopped dried apricots

¼ cup apricot preserves

Serves 12

12 turkey steaks

9 tablespoons flour

1½ teaspoons salt

1½ teaspoons cumin

9 tablespoons olive oil

3 cups apricot nectar

1½ cups chopped dried apricots

¾ cup apricot preserves

1. Lightly pound turkey steaks to flatten slightly. On shallow plate, combine flour, salt, and cumin and coat turkey steaks with mixture on both sides. Heat olive oil in heavy skillet and cook steaks in batches until browned on both sides, about 4 to 5 minutes per batch. Remove steaks as they are browned.

2. Return steaks to skillet and add apricot nectar and chopped dried apricots. Bring to a boil, reduce heat, and simmer for 8 to 12 minutes, until turkey is thoroughly cooked. Cool in ice-water bath or refrigerator; then pour into zipper-lock bag. Attach small bags with apricot preserves, label bags, and freeze.

3. To thaw and reheat: Thaw overnight in refrigerator. Place steaks, sauce, and apricot preserves in heavy skillet. Bring to a simmer over medium heat and cook until steaks are thoroughly heated and glazed, about 8 to 10 minutes.

Spicy Turkey Meatballs

Try an exotic rice with these spicy meatballs; basmati or jasmine would be wonderful. To serve immediately simply serve meatballs and sauce when meat is thoroughly cooked.

Serves 4

1 pound ground turkey

1 egg

½ cup minced onion

1 jalapeno pepper, minced

¼ cup tomato juice

½ cup dried bread crumbs

½ teaspoon salt

1 teaspoon crushed red pepper flakes

2 tablespoons olive oil

4 cloves garlic, minced

2 cups Chicken Broth

1 (10-ounce) jar Alfredo sauce

1 cup shredded pepper jack cheese

Serves 12

3 pounds ground turkey

3 eggs

1½ cups minced onion

3 jalapeno peppers, minced

¾ cup tomato juice

1½ cups dried bread crumbs

1½ teaspoons salt

1 teaspoon crushed red pepper flakes

6 tablespoons olive oil

12 cloves garlic, minced

6 cups Chicken Broth

3 (10-ounce) jars Alfredo sauce

3 cups shredded pepper jack cheese

1. In large bowl, combine turkey, egg, onion, jalapeno pepper, tomato juice, bread crumbs, salt, and red pepper flakes and blend well. Form into 24 (or 72) meatballs. Heat olive oil in large skillet and brown meatballs, in batches, on all sides, about 4 to 5 minutes per batch.

2. Drain excess fat from skillet and add garlic. Cook and stir for 1 to 2 minutes. Return meatballs to skillet along with chicken broth. Bring to a boil, reduce heat, cover pan, and simmer meatballs for 15 to 20 minutes until thoroughly cooked. Stir Alfredo sauce and cheese into skillet and simmer 1 to 2 minutes to blend flavors. Cool in ice-water bath or refrigerator. Pack into zipper-lock bags, label, seal, and freeze.

3. To thaw and reheat: Thaw meatballs and sauce overnight in refrigerator. Place in a heavy skillet and add ¼cup water if the mixture looks dry. Bring to a boil and simmer for 10 to 15 minutes, until meatballs are thoroughly heated.

Italian Turkey Sauce

You can use ground turkey breast or a combination of dark and light meat in this easy sauce. To serve immediately cook spaghetti as directed on package and serve sauce over pasta.

Serves 4

1 pound ground turkey

1 onion, chopped

2 cups mushrooms, chopped

2 tablespoons olive oil

½ teaspoon salt

1 teaspoon Italian seasoning

1 (14-ounce) jar pasta sauce

1 (14-ounce) can diced tomatoes, undrained

1 cup grated Parmesan cheese

1 (8-ounce) package spaghetti

Serves 12

3 pounds ground turkey

3 onions, chopped

6 cups mushrooms, chopped

6 tablespoons olive oil

1½ teaspoons salt

1 tablespoon Italian seasoning

3 (14-ounce) jars pasta sauce

3 (14-ounce) cans diced tomatoes, undrained

3 cups grated Parmesan cheese

3 (8-ounce) packages spaghetti

1. In heavy skillet, sauté turkey, onion, and mushrooms in olive oil until turkey is browned, stirring to break up meat. Drain if necessary; then add remaining ingredients except cheese and pasta. Simmer for 5 to 8 minutes, until turkey is thoroughly cooked and flavors are blended.

2. Cool sauce in an ice-water bath or in refrigerator. Pack into zipper-lock bags and attach small bags with Parmesan cheese; label, seal and freeze. Reserve pasta in the pantry.

3. To thaw and reheat: Thaw sauce overnight in refrigerator. Pour into a heavy skillet and bring to a boil. Reduce heat and simmer for 8 to 10 minutes, until thoroughly heated. Cook spaghetti according to package directions, drain, and serve sauce over pasta. Sprinkle each serving with cheese.

Stuffed Turkey Tenderloins

The unusual sweet and spicy filling that stuffs these tenderloins is delicious. To serve without freezing, just serve the rolls after they are thoroughly cooked.

Serves 4

2 turkey tenderloins

1 teaspoon salt

1 teaspoon white pepper

½ cup golden raisins

½ cup dried fruit bits

1 (3-ounce) package cream cheese

2 tablespoons honey mustard

1 tablespoon honey

1 cup dried bread crumbs

Serves 12

6 turkey tenderloins

1 tablespoon salt

1 teaspoon white pepper

½ cups golden raisins

1½ cups dried fruit bits

3 (3-ounce) packages cream cheese

6 tablespoons honey mustard

3 tablespoons honey

3 cups dried bread crumbs

1. Cut turkey tenderloins in half crosswise to make four pieces. Cut slit inside of each piece and spread turkey pieces open. Sprinkle with salt and pepper. In small bowl, combine raisins, dried fruit, cream cheese, and honey mustard and mix well. Divide this mixture among turkey pieces and fold to enclose filling. Use toothpicks to secure edges.

2. Preheat oven to 400°F. Coat tenderloins with honey and roll in bread crumbs. Place in 9″ × 13″ baking pan and bake at 350°F for 40 to 45 minutes, turning once, until internal temperature registers

170°F. Cool rolls in refrigerator, then wrap individually in freezer wrap and place in zipper-lock bags. Label, seal, and freeze.

3. To thaw and reheat: Thaw overnight in refrigerator. Preheat oven to 400°F. Place turkey rolls in 9″ × 13″ baking pan and bake at 400°F for 18 to 25 minutes or until thoroughly heated and bread crumb coating is crisp.

Tex Mex Pork Casserole

To serve without freezing, add kidney beans to casserole after 90 minutes of cooking.

Simmer another 20 to 30 minutes, until sauce is thickened.

Serves 6–8

2 pounds boneless pork chops

1 cup Beef Broth

¼ cup red wine vinegar

½ cup red wine

2 cloves garlic, minced

1 jalapeno pepper, minced

2 tablespoons honey

1 teaspoon pepper

2 tablespoons olive oil

1 tablespoon butter

1 onion, chopped

½ cup Beef Broth

½ cup taco sauce

2 (16-ounce) cans kidney beans

Serves 18–24

6 pounds boneless pork chops

3 cups Beef Broth

¾ cup red wine vinegar

1½ cups red wine

6 cloves garlic, minced

3 jalapeno peppers, minced

6 tablespoons honey

1 teaspoon pepper

6 tablespoons olive oil

3 tablespoons butter

3 onions, chopped

1½ cups Beef Broth

1½ cups taco sauce

6 (16-ounce) cans kidney beans

1. Cut pork chops into 1-inch cubes. In large bowl, combine the first quantity of broth, vinegar, red wine, garlic, peppers, honey, and pepper. Add pork cubes to this mixture, cover, and refrigerate overnight.

2. Drain pork, reserving marinade. Pat pork dry with paper towels. Heat olive oil and butter in heavy skillet and add pork in batches. Cook, stirring frequently, for 4 minutes per batch, removing pork from the pan as it browns. When all pork is browned, return to

skillet along with reserved marinade and onion, beef broth, and taco sauce. Bring to a boil, cover pan, reduce heat,

and simmer mixture for 1½ hours until pork is tender. Cool mixture in an ice-water bath or in refrigerator. Pour mixture into zipper-lock bags, label, and freeze. Reserve kidney beans in the pantry.

3. To thaw and reheat: Thaw overnight in refrigerator. Pour mixture into a heavy skillet and bring to a boil. Drain kidney beans, rinse, drain again, and add to skillet. Reduce heat, cover, and simmer casserole for 15 to 20 minutes, until thoroughly heated.

Citrus Pork Stew

To serve without freezing, serve stew after pork is thoroughly cooked.

Serves 6–8

2 pounds boneless pork shoulder

1 teaspoon salt

1 teaspoon white pepper

1 teaspoon grated orange rind

¼ cup flour

¼ cup olive oil

3 tablespoons butter

1 onion, chopped

5 cups Chicken Broth

1 cup of orange juice

1 cup white wine

1 (9-ounce) bag baby carrots

1 cup chopped fennel

Serves 18–24

6 pounds boneless pork shoulder

1 tablespoon salt

1 teaspoon white pepper

1 tablespoon grated orange rind

¾ cup flour

¾ cup olive oil

9 tablespoons butter

3 onions, chopped

15 cups Chicken Broth

3 cups orange juice

3 cups white wine

3 (9-ounce) bags baby carrots

3 cups chopped fennel

1. Trim excess fat from pork and cut into 1-inch cubes. On shallow plate, combine salt, pepper, orange rind, and flour. Toss pork in this mixture to coat. In heavy skillet, heat olive oil and butter. Add coated pork cubes in batches, and cook until browned, stirring occasionally.

Remove pork from pan as it browns.

2. Add onion to pan and cook until crisp-tender, 3 to 4 minutes. Return pork to pan along with all remaining ingredients. Bring to a

boil; then reduce heat, cover pan, and simmer the stew for 1½ hours, until pork is thoroughly cooked. Cool stew in ice-water bath or in refrigerator. Pour into rigid containers, label, seal, and freeze.

3. To thaw and reheat: Thaw stew overnight in refrigerator. Pour into large saucepan and bring to a boil. Simmer over medium-low heat for 15 to 20 minutes, until thoroughly heated.

Pork and Tomato Farfalle

To serve without freezing, marinate pork in the refrigerator for 2 hours. Cook sauce as directed and let simmer while sautéing pork slices. Pour sauce over pork and simmer for 10 minutes; then add milk.

Serves 6

1 pound pork tenderloin

½ teaspoon salt

1 teaspoon pepper

4 cloves garlic, minced

2 tablespoons olive oil

1 onion, chopped

1 (14-ounce) can diced tomatoes, undrained

1 (8-ounce) can tomato paste

2 tablespoons sugar

½ teaspoon dried basil leaves

½ teaspoon dried thyme leaves

3 cups farfalle pasta

½ cup evaporated milk

Serves 18

3 pounds pork tenderloin

1½ teaspoons salt

1 teaspoon pepper

12 cloves garlic, minced

6 tablespoons olive oil

3 onions, chopped

3 (14-ounce) cans diced tomatoes, undrained

3 (8-ounce) cans tomato paste

6 tablespoons sugar

1½ teaspoons dried basil leaves

1½ teaspoons dried thyme leaves

9 cups farfalle pasta

1½ cups evaporated milk

1. Slice pork tenderloin crosswise into ¼-inch slices. In small bowl, combine salt, pepper, and garlic. Using the back of the spoon, crush garlic into spices until paste forms. Rub this paste on the pork tenderloin slices. Place pork in a zipper-lock bag and set in refrigerator.

2. In heavy skillet, heat olive oil and cook onion until crisp-tender. Add undrained tomatoes, tomato paste, sugar, basil, and thyme. Bring to a boil, reduce heat, cover pan, and simmer for 15 minutes to blend flavors. Cool sauce in an ice-water bath or refrigerator.

Pour into zipper-lock bag, attach to pork bag, label, and freeze. Reserve pasta and evaporated milk in the pantry.

3. To thaw and reheat: Thaw pork and sauce overnight in refrigerator. Heat 1 tablespoon olive oil in large skillet. Add pork slices and cook, turning once, until pork is browned, about 5 minutes.

Add tomato sauce to pan and bring to a boil. Simmer, covered, for 15 to 20 minutes, until pork is tender, then add evaporated milk and simmer 3 minutes longer. Cook pasta as directed on package, drain, and serve with pork.

Pineapple Pork Chops

To serve without freezing, marinate chops in refrigerator for 4 to 8 hours, then cook as directed below. Be sure to boil marinade before serving.

Serves 6

6 (¾-inch-thick) boneless pork chops

1 teaspoon salt

1 teaspoon white pepper

2 cloves garlic, chopped

1 (8-ounce) can pineapple tidbits, undrained

1 tablespoon honey

2 teaspoons grated ginger root

½ cup pineapple preserves

Serves 18

18 (¾-inch-thick) boneless pork chops

1 tablespoon salt

1 teaspoon white pepper

6 cloves garlic, chopped

3 (8-ounce) cans pineapple tidbits, undrained

3 tablespoons honey

2 tablespoons grated ginger root

1½ cups pineapple preserves

1. Trim excess fat from pork chops and sprinkle with salt and pepper. Combine all remaining ingredients in a large zipper-lock bag and add pork chops. Seal bag and knead to distribute sauce. Label bag and freeze.

2. To thaw and cook: Thaw overnight in the refrigerator. Remove chops from marinade and broil or grill 4 to 6 inches from heat source for 12 to 15 minutes, until pork chops are no longer pink in center. Place marinade in small saucepan and bring to a boil. Boil for 3 minutes, stirring frequently. Serve marinade with chops.

Honey Mustard Pork Chops

These easy pork chops are packed full of flavor. To serve without freezing, marinate pork chops in refrigerator for 4 to 8 hours, then broil as directed.

Serves 6

¼ cup mustard

¼ cup honey

2 tablespoons apple cider vinegar

1 teaspoon pepper

¼ teaspoon garlic powder

½ teaspoon dried thyme

½ teaspoon dried marjoram

6 boneless pork loin chops

Serves 18

¾ cup mustard

¾ cup honey

6 tablespoons apple cider vinegar

1 teaspoon pepper

¾ teaspoon garlic powder

½ teaspoons dried thyme

½ teaspoons dried marjoram

18 boneless pork loin chops

1. In zipper-lock bag, combine all ingredients except pork chops and squish the bag to mix. Add pork chops, seal bag, label, and freeze.

2. To thaw and reheat: Thaw overnight in refrigerator. Broil pork chops 4 to 6 inches from heat source for 18 to 20 minutes, turning once, until internal temperature registers 160°F. Discard any remaining marinade.

Apple Glazed Pork Roast

To serve without freezing, when pork reaches 160°F, remove from oven, cover with foil, and let stand for 10 minutes. Thinly slice and serve with sauce.

Serves 6–8

1 (3-pound) boneless pork sirloin roast

1 teaspoon salt

1 teaspoon pepper

2 tablespoons olive oil

3 cloves garlic, minced

1 cup apple cider

½ cup apple jelly

2 tablespoons apple cider vinegar

2 tablespoons brown sugar

Serves 18–24

3 (3-pound) boneless pork sirloin roasts

1 tablespoon salt

1 teaspoon pepper

6 tablespoons olive oil

9 cloves garlic, minced

3 cups apple cider

1½ cups apple jelly

6 tablespoons apple cider vinegar

6 tablespoons brown sugar

1. Preheat oven to 400°F. Trim excess fat from roast. Sprinkle on all sides with salt and pepper. In heavy skillet, brown roast on all sides in olive oil over medium heat. Remove pork from pan and add remaining ingredients to the skillet. Cook and stir over medium heat until sugar dissolves and mixture comes to a boil.

2. Place pork in roasting pan and roast at 400°F for 30 minutes. Then pour apple cider mixture over all and roast 35 to 45 minutes longer, basting occasionally with sauce, until instant-read thermometer measures 160°F. Cool pork and sauce in refrigerator. Thinly slice pork and place in zipper-lock bag along with sauce. Seal bag, label, and freeze.

3. To thaw and reheat: Thaw overnight in refrigerator. Place pork and sauce in heavy skillet and bring to a simmer over medium heat. Cook for 4 to 5 minutes, until pork is thoroughly heated.

BBQ Ribs

Experience a new variation on your favorite homemade or store-bought barbecue sauce in this recipe. To serve immediately, cook ribs as directed, basting frequently with sauce, until they are very tender.

Serves 4

4 pounds meaty pork short ribs

1 teaspoon salt

1 teaspoon pepper

1 onion, chopped

5 cloves garlic, chopped

2 tablespoons olive oil

½ cup honey

½ cup barbecue sauce

1 tablespoon mustard

1 cup Beef Broth

Serves 12

12 pounds meaty pork short ribs

1 tablespoon salt

1 teaspoon pepper

3 onions, chopped

15 cloves garlic, chopped

6 tablespoons olive oil

1½ cups honey

1½ cups barbecue sauce

3 tablespoons mustard

3 cups Beef Broth

1. Preheat oven to 400°F. Sprinkle ribs with salt and pepper and place in baking pan. Roast ribs, uncovered, for 1 hour.

2. While ribs are roasting, in a heavy skillet, sauté onion and garlic in olive oil until tender. Add remaining ingredients and bring to a boil. Reduce heat and simmer for 15 to 20 minutes, stirring frequently, until slightly thickened.

3. After ribs are roasted, drain fat from pan. Pour sauce over ribs. Reduce oven temperature to 350°F and roast ribs for another 80 to 95 minutes, basting occasionally with sauce, until ribs are very tender. Cool ribs in refrigerator. Pack into zipper-lock bags with sauce, label packages, and freeze.

4. To thaw and reheat: Thaw ribs overnight in refrigerator. Place ribs on baking pan and cover with sauce. Bake at 350°F for 20 to 25 minutes, until ribs are glazed and thoroughly heated.

Olive Tarts

To serve immediately, sprinkle with cheese and bake at 400°F for 10 to 12 minutes or until pastry is golden brown, a filling is set, and cheese is melted and beginning to brown.

Makes 24

1 onion, chopped

2 cloves garlic, minced

½ cup chopped mushrooms

1 tablespoon olive oil

½ cup sliced black olives

½ cup sliced green olives

½ teaspoon dried thyme leaves

2 sheets frozen puff pastry, thawed

1 cup shredded Gouda cheese

Makes 72

3 onions, chopped

6 cloves garlic, minced

1½ cups chopped mushrooms

3 tablespoons olive oil

1½cups sliced black olives

1½ cups sliced green olives

1½ teaspoons dried thyme leaves

6 sheets frozen puff pastry, thawed

3 cups shredded Cuda cheese

1. Preheat oven to 400°F. In heavy skillet, sauté onion, garlic, and mushrooms in olive oil until tender. Remove from heat and add olives and thyme.

2. Gently roll puff pastry dough with rolling pin until ¼-inch thick. Using a 3-inch cookie cutter, cut 24 circles from pastry. Line muffin cups with dough.

3. Place a spoonful of filling in each pastry-lined cup. Bake at 400°F for 10 to 12 minutes or until

crust is golden brown and filling is set.

4. Remove from muffin cups and cool on wire rack. Flash freeze; when frozen solid, pack tarts into zipper-lock bags. Attach zipper-lock bag filled with shredded cheese; label and freeze.

5. To thaw and reheat: Thaw tarts in a single layer overnight in refrigerator. Top each tart with

cheese and bake at 400°F for 5 to 6 minutes or until hot and cheese is melted.

Shrimp Quiches

To serve immediately, bake quiches at 375°F for 15 to 18 minutes, until filling is set and pastry is browned. Let cool for 10 minutes before serving.

Makes 36

2 9-inch Pie Crusts

½ cup chopped leek, rinsed

1 tablespoon olive oil

2 eggs

½ cup cream

1 (6-ounce) can tiny shrimp, drained

½ teaspoon dried marjoram leaves

½ teaspoon salt teaspoon pepper

¾ cup shredded Havarti cheese

Makes 108

6 9-inch Pie Crusts

1½ cups chopped leek, rinsed

3 tablespoons olive oil

6 eggs

1½ cups cream

3 (6-ounce) cans tiny shrimp, drained

1½ teaspoons dried marjoram leaves

½ teaspoons salt

1 teaspoon pepper

2¼ cups shredded Havarti cheese

1. Using a 2-inch cookie cutter, cut 36 rounds from pie crusts. Place each in a 1¾-inch mini muffin cup, pressing to bottom and sides. Set aside.

2. Sauté leek in olive oil until tender. Beat eggs with cream in medium bowl. Add drained shrimp, cooked leek, marjoram, salt, and pepper, and mix well.

3. Sprinkle 1 teaspoon cheese into each muffin cup and fill cups with shrimp mixture. Bake at
375°F for 15 to 18 minutes or until pastry is golden and filling is set. Cool in refrigerator until
cold, then freeze.

4. Freeze in a single layer on the baking sheet. When frozen solid, pack in rigid containers, using waxed paper to separate layers. Label and freeze.

5. To reheat: Place frozen quiches on baking sheet and bake at 375°F for 8 to 11 minutes or until
hot.

Egg Rolls

To serve immediately, fry in peanut oil at 375°F for 2 to 3 minutes, until golden brown. To make a dipping sauce, mix 3 tablespoons soy sauce with 1 teaspoon sugar, 1 tablespoon mustard, and 1 tablespoon vinegar.

Makes 24

½ pound ground pork

½ pound ground shrimp

1 carrot, shredded

2 cloves garlic, minced

1 bunch green onions, finely chopped

1 cup shredded Napa cabbage

2 tablespoons soy sauce

1 tablespoon oyster sauce

2 tablespoons cornstarch 1 tablespoon water

1 package egg roll wrappers

3 cups peanut oil

Makes 72

1½ pounds ground pork

1½ pounds ground shrimp

3 carrots, shredded

6 cloves garlic, minced

3 bunches green onions, finely chopped

3 cups shredded Napa cabbage

6 tablespoons soy sauce

3 tablespoons oyster sauce

6 tablespoons cornstarch

3 tablespoons water

3 packages egg roll wrappers

3 cups peanut oil

1. In a large skillet, brown ground pork until almost done. Add ground shrimp, carrot, and garlic; cook and stir for 4 to 6 minutes or until pork is cooked. Remove from heat, drain well, and add green onions, cabbage, soy sauce, and oyster sauce.

2. Combine cornstarch and water in a small bowl and blend well.

3. To form egg rolls, place one wrapper, point-side down, on work surface. Place 1 tablespoon filling 1 inch from corner. Brush all edges of the egg roll wrapper with cornstarch mixture. Fold point over filling, then fold in sides and roll up egg roll, using cornstarch mixture to seal as necessary.

4. At this point, egg rolls may be flash frozen, or you can flash freeze them after frying. Once frozen, pack, label, and freeze in rigid containers.

5. To reheat untried egg rolls: Fry the frozen rolls in peanut oil heated to 375°F for 2 to 3 minutes, turning once, or until deep golden brown.

To reheat fried egg rolls: Place frozen egg rolls on the baking sheet. Bake at 375°F for 8 to 10 minutes or until crisp and hot.

Beefy Mini Pies

Include these pies in an appetizer buffet, or serve them to guests before dinner with a glass of red wine. To serve immediately, bake at 350°F for 7 to 9 minutes; serve hot.

Makes 24

1 (10-ounce) package refrigerated flaky dinner rolls

½ pound ground beef

1 small onion, chopped

2 cloves garlic, minced

1 cup shredded Colby cheese

2 eggs

½ cup half-and-half

½ teaspoon dried dill weed

Makes 72

3 (10-ounce) packages refrigerated flaky dinner rolls

1½ pounds ground beef

3 small onions, chopped

6 cloves garlic, minced

3 cups shredded Colby cheese

6 eggs

1½ cups half-and-half

1½ teaspoons dried dill weed

1. Preheat oven to 350°F. Remove rolls from package and divide each roll into 3 rounds. Place

each round into a 3-inch muffin cup; press firmly onto bottom and upsides.

2. In a heavy skillet, cook ground beef with onion and garlic until beef is done. Drain well. Place 1 tablespoon beef mixture into each dough-lined muffin cup. Sprinkle cheese over beef mixture. In a small bowl, beat together eggs, half-and-half, and dill weed. Spoon this mixture over beef in

muffin cups, making sure not to overfill cups.

3. Bake at 350°F for 10 to 13 minutes or until filling is puffed and set. Flash freeze in a single layer on the baking sheet. When frozen solid, wrap, label, and freeze.

4. To thaw and reheat: Thaw pies in a single layer in the refrigerator overnight. Bake at 350°F for 7 to 9 minutes or until hot.

Olive Puffs

You can make these little puffs with any type of stuffed olive and any type of cheese. To serve immediately bake at 400°F for 10 to 12 minutes.

Makes 30

5 tablespoons butter, softened

1 (3-ounce) package cream cheese, softened

1½ cups grated sharp Cheddar cheese

1 teaspoon Worcestershire sauce

¾ cup flour

teaspoon pepper

30 garlic-stuffed olives

Makes 90

15 tablespoons butter, softened

3 (3-ounce) packages cream cheese, softened

4½ cups grated sharp Cheddar cheese

1 tablespoon Worcestershire sauce

2¼ cups flour

1 teaspoon pepper

90 garlic-stuffed olives

1. In medium bowl, combine butter, cream cheese, and Cheddar cheese. Cream well until blended. Add Worcestershire sauce and mix until blended. Add flour and pepper and mix to form dough.

2. Form dough around each olive, covering olive completely. Flash freeze in a single layer on baking sheets, then package in zipper-lock bags. Label bag and freeze.

3. To reheat: Place frozen puffs on the baking sheet. Bake at 400°F for 10 to 12 minutes or until hot,

puffed, and golden brown.

Nutty Parmesan Sticks

To serve immediately, let cool after baking and serve with a soft cheese dip. Store sticks in airtight container at room temperature.

Makes 36

1 package frozen puff pastry sheets, thawed

½ cup ground almonds

½ cup grated Parmesan cheese

teaspoon cayenne pepper

Makes 72

3 packages frozen puff pastry sheets, thawed

1½ cups ground almonds

1½ cups grated Parmesan cheese

teaspoon cayenne pepper

1. Preheat oven to 375°F. In a small bowl, combine almonds, cheese, and pepper; blend well.

Sprinkle half of this mixture over work surface and cover with one sheet puff pastry. Using a rolling pin, gently press pastry into cheese mixture. Turn pastry over and press cheese mixture into the other side of the pastry. Repeat with other half of cheese mixture and second sheet of puff

pastry.

2. Using pastry cutter or sharp knife, cut pastry into ½-inch strips. Place on parchment paper- or

foil-lined baking sheets, twisting each strip several times. Bake at 375°F for 10 to 15 minutes or

until browned and crisp, being careful not to burn sticks. Remove from baking sheet and cool

completely on wire racks. Pack carefully into rigid containers, separating layers with waxed

paper. Label containers and freeze.

3. To thaw and reheat: Thaw sticks at room temperature and serve, or carefully place frozen sticks on baking sheet and bake at 350°F for 4 to 5 minutes or until hot.

Shrimp and Artichoke Puffs

To serve these delicate and delicious puffs immediately, bake at 400°F for 7 to 9

minutes or until hot and bubbling, then offer them to your guests with white wine.

Makes about 24

6 slices whole-wheat bread

2 shallots, chopped

1 tablespoon olive oil

½ pound cooked shrimp

1 (10-ounce) package frozen artichoke hearts, thawed

1 (3-ounce) package cream cheese, softened

1 cup shredded Cuda cheese

½ cup mayonnaise

1 tablespoon lemon juice

1 teaspoon dried basil leaves

Makes about 72

18 slices whole-wheat bread

6 shallots, chopped

3 tablespoons olive oil

1½ pounds cooked shrimp

3 (10-ounce) packages frozen artichoke hearts, thawed

3 (3-ounce) packages cream cheese, softened

3 cups shredded Gouda cheese

1½ cups mayonnaise

3 tablespoons lemon juice

1 tablespoon dried basil leaves

1. Preheat oven to 300°F. Using a 2-inch cookie cutter, cut rounds from bread slices. Place rounds on a baking sheet and bake at 300°F for 7 to 9 minutes, or until crisp, turning once. Remove from oven and cool on wire racks.

2. In a heavy skillet, cook shallots in olive oil over medium heat until tender. Remove from heat.

Chop shrimp and add to skillet along with thawed, drained, and chopped artichoke hearts. Add

both cheeses, mayonnaise, lemon juice, and basil; stir well to blend.

3. Spoon 1 tablespoon shrimp mixture onto each bread round, covering the top and mounding the

filling. Flash freeze on baking sheets. When frozen solid, pack in rigid containers, with waxed

paper between layers. Label puffs and freeze.

4. To reheat: Place frozen puffs on a baking sheet and bake at 400°F for 10 to 12 minutes or until

topping is hot and bubbling.

Stuffed Mushrooms

Lemon juice prevents the mushrooms from darkening during freezing and adds a fresh flavor. To serve immediately, bake filled mushrooms at 375°F for 8 to 10 minutes or until hot and cheese is melted.

Makes 30

30 large mushrooms

2 tablespoons lemon juice

2 tablespoons olive oil

1 onion, finely chopped

1 tablespoon olive oil

1 Cranny Smith apple, peeled and finely chopped

½ cup chopped walnuts

1 cup cubed Havarti cheese

½ teaspoon salt

1 teaspoon pepper

Makes 90

90 large mushrooms

6 tablespoons lemon juice

6 tablespoons olive oil

3 onions, finely chopped

3 tablespoons olive oil

3 Cranny Smith apples, peeled and finely chopped

1½ cups chopped walnuts

3 cups cubed Havarti cheese

½ teaspoons salt

1 teaspoon pepper

1. Preheat oven to 375ºF. Remove stems from mushrooms; chop stems and set aside. Combine

lemon juice and olive oil in a small bowl and dip mushroom caps into this mixture. Place

mushroom caps upside down on baking sheet and bake at 375ºF for 6 to 8 minutes, or until

slightly softened. Remove from oven and cool.

2. In a heavy skillet, sauté onion and chopped mushroom stems in olive oil until tender. Add

chopped apple and walnuts; mix well. Remove from heat and cool for 20 minutes. Stir in cheese,

salt, and pepper.

3. Stuff mushrooms with filling mixture, smoothing the top of filling. Flash freeze mushrooms on baking sheets. When frozen, pack mushrooms in rigid containers, with waxed paper separating layers. Label mushrooms and freeze.

4. To reheat: Bake frozen mushrooms at 375ºF for 15 to 18 minutes or until mushrooms are hot and beginning to brown and cheese is melted.

Mini Crab Cakes

Serve these crab cakes with mayonnaise blended with cilantro and Romano cheese. To serve immediately, fry until golden and hot, turning once, about 3 to 5 minutes on each side.

Makes about 24

1 pound canned lump crabmeat

1 cup fresh cilantro leaves

½ cup chopped walnuts

½ cup grated Romano cheese

2 tablespoons olive oil

½ cup dried bread crumbs

½ cup mayonnaise

¼ cup minced green onions

3 tablespoons olive oil

Makes about 72

3 pounds canned lump crabmeat

3 cups fresh cilantro leaves

1½ cups chopped walnuts

1½ cups grated Romano cheese

6 tablespoons olive oil

1½ cups dried bread crumbs

1½ cups mayonnaise

¾ A cup minced green onions

9 tablespoons olive oil

1. Drain crabmeat well and pick over to remove any cartilage. Set aside in large bowl. In food processor or blender, combine cilantro, walnuts, cheese, and 2 tablespoons olive oil (6 tablespoons for triple batch). Process or blend until mixture forms a paste. Stir into crabmeat.

2. Add bread crumbs, mayonnaise, and green onions to crab mixture. Stir to combine. Form into 2-inch patties about ½-inch thick. Flash freeze on the baking sheet. When frozen solid, pack crab cakes in rigid containers, with waxed paper between the layers. Label crab cakes and freeze. Reserve remaining olive oil in the pantry.

3. To thaw and reheat: Thaw crab cakes in refrigerator overnight. Heat 3 tablespoons olive oil (9 for a triple batch) in large, heavy skillet over medium heat. Fry crab cakes until golden and hot, turning once, about 3 to 5 minutes on each side.

Italian Pork Skewers

These skewers are tender and full of flavor. To serve immediately, marinate for 2 to 3 hours, then cook over grill or broil until done.

Serves 6–8

2 pounds pork tenderloin

¼ cup balsamic vinegar

¼ cup olive oil

¼ cup finely minced onion

1 teaspoon dried Italian seasoning

½ teaspoon salt

1 teaspoon pepper

Serves 18–24

6 pounds pork tenderloin

¾ cup balsamic vinegar

¾ cup olive oil

¾ cup finely minced onion

1 tablespoon dried Italian seasoning

1½ teaspoons salt

1 teaspoon pepper

1. Trim excess fat from tenderloin. Cut pork, on a slant, into ¼-inch-thick slices, each about 4 inches long. In large bowl, combine remaining ingredients and mix well with wire whisk. Add tenderloin slices and mix gently to coat. Cover and refrigerate for 2 to 3 hours. Meanwhile, soak 8-inch wooden skewers in cold water.

2. Remove pork from marinade and thread onto soaked skewers. Flash freeze on the baking sheet in a single layer. When frozen solid, pack skewers in rigid containers, with layers separated by waxed paper. Label skewers and freeze.

3. To thaw and reheat: Thaw overnight in refrigerator. Cook skewers 4 to 6 inches from medium coals on grill, or broil 4 to 6 inches from heat source, for about 4 to 6 minutes or until cooked (160°F on an instant-read thermometer), turning once.

CPSIA information can be obtained
at www.ICGtesting.com
Printed in the USA
BVHW071149021120
592330BV00008B/412